QUESTIONS AND ANSWERS FOR PHYSICIANS

SIR HENRY WELLCOME ASIAN STUDIES

EDITED BY

LAWRENCE I. CONRAD
DOMINIK WUJASTYK
PAUL U. UNSCHULD

VOLUME 3

QUESTIONS AND ANSWERS FOR PHYSICIANS

A Medieval Arabic Study Manual by ʿAbd al-ʿAzīz al-Sulamī

TRANSLATED, EDITED, AND WITH AN INTRODUCTION BY

GARY LEISER
AND
NOURY AL-KHALEDY

BRILL
LEIDEN · BOSTON
2004

This book is printed on acid-free paper.

Library of Congress Cataloging-in-Publication Data

Al-Sulami, ʿAbd al-ʿAziz.
Questions and answers for physicians : a medieval Arabic study manual by ʿAbd al-ʿAziz Al-Sulami / translated, edited, and with an introduction by Gary Leiser and Noury Al-Khaledy.
p. cm. — (The Sir Henry Wellcome Asian series)
ISBN 90-04-13671-1
1. Medicine, Arab—History. 2. Medicine, Medieval. 3. Medicine--Study and teaching. I. Leiser, Gary, 1946- II. Al-Khaledy, Noury. III. Title. IV. Series.

R143.A439 2003
610—dc22

2003065334

ISSN 1570-1484
ISBN 90 04 13671 1

PRINTED IN THE NETHERLANDS

In Memory of

Martin Levey
and
Michael Dols

CONTENTS

PREFACE

In 1977, while doing research on medical education in the medieval Middle East, I came across a manuscript with the intriguing title *Imtiḥān al-alibbā' li-kāffat al-aṭibbā'* ["The Experts' Examination for All Physicians"] in a catalogue of Arabic manuscripts in Vienna. I subsequently acquired a copy of this work on microfilm. After briefly examining its contents, I happened to mention it to one of my former undergraduate professors of Arabic, Noury Al-Khaledy. Because of his interest in pharmacology and my interest in pedagogy and because, above all, I had discovered no other work quite like it surviving from the medieval Muslim world, he suggested that we edit and translate the manuscript. I agreed and we soon made a very preliminary reading and translation of it. Shortly thereafter, we located a second copy of this work in Cairo and a third in Bursa. We then had the resources to prepare a proper collated edition of the text. My professional peregrinations, however, and Prof. Al-Khaledy's university duties and then his retirement and responsibilities to a private firm prevented us from promptly carrying out this project. Over the years, we managed to publish only a description of the work in a Turkish scholarly journal. In 1992, Prof. Al-Khaledy's health began to fail and on 19 October 1995 he passed away. Meanwhile, I had assembled all the materials that we had collected and began to review those parts of the translation that I had revised since our first draft. And thanks to modern computer technology, which now allows one to produce an Arabic text at home, I was able to edit the work and finally prepare a complete translation. This translation, I hasten to add, has benefitted in no small way from the expert criticism of Lawrence Conrad at the University of Hamburg. It is with deep regret that I was not able to finish this task before Prof. Al-Khaledy's death.

A few words are in order here about Noury Al-Khaledy, known simply as Noury to his friends, and his remarkable career and contributions to the teaching of Arabic in the United States. Noury gave his birth date as 1 February 1918, although he was not absolutely certain. Born in Damascus, he was a descendant of a famous Arabian tribe, the Banī Khālid of the Syrian Desert. Indeed, although his mother was Circassian, he spent his early childhood as a bedouin. Nevertheless, he attended high school at North Syria School for Boys in Aleppo and went on to graduate from Aleppo College, which was run by the Congregational and Presbyterian churches, in 1941. Between 1943 and 1945 he was a regional inspector in various parts of Syria. In 1946 he was the regional director of Jazīra, primarily with respect to the distribution of wheat. In the same year, he became head of the legal department of North Syria. In 1947, he received a bachelors degree from the American University in Beirut and later, in 1950, a law degree from the Syrian University in Damascus.

Around 1940, Noury had joined the secular Syrian National Party, more widely known as the Parti Populaire Syrien, or PPS. An increasingly popular member, he rose in the ranks to become head of the party's two branches in Damascus and Aleppo in the early 1950s. On 22 April 1955, 'Adnān al-Malkī, the Deputy Chief of Staff of the Syrian Army, was assassinated by a soldier who happened to be a member of the PPS. The Communist and Ba'th parties then used this as an excuse to eliminate the PPS—being neither Socialist nor pan-Arab but nationalist and moderately pro-Western—from Syrian public life. Forewarned of the coming roundup of PPS leaders, Noury went into hiding in Syria for more than four months. Finally, in late 1955, he fled in disguise to Iskenderun, Turkey. His fiancée later joined him there, and after they were married they went to Gaziantep to stay with her Circassian relatives.

In 1957, through his contacts at Aleppo College, and with the express permission of Secretary of State John Foster Dulles, he went to New York with an ecumenical fellowship in religious studies at Union Theological Seminary. Between 1958 and 1960, he was a research assistant in the Department of Oriental Studies at Princeton. Senator Margaret Chase Smith from Maine helped arrange funding for his position. At Princeton he met Farhat Ziadeh and collaborated with him on the production of *A Reader in Modern Literary Arabic*. He also met Martin Levey, who was at the Institute for Advanced Study, and together they later published *The Medical Formulary of al-Samarqandī*.

In late 1960, Noury moved to Portland, Oregon where he joined the Department of Foreign Languages at Portland State College, which was founded in 1946 to provide educational opportunies for veterans of World War II. In fact, he had been recruited to create a program in teaching Arabic in the college's Middle East Studies Center (MESC). Established in 1959 through the efforts of Frederick Cox, its first director, it was one of twelve such centers in the United States supported by the US Office of Education and the only one devoted exclusively to undergraduate education. As a result of the dynamism of the MESC, through the efforts of Cox and Al-Khaledy in particular, the young college became almost synonomous with Middle Eastern Studies in the 1960s and 70s, especially instruction in Arabic. In 1961 the MESC was designated one of the ten federal depositories to receive library materials from the United Arab Republic under Public Law 480. This allowed the college library to build one of the best Arabic collections in the western United States.

In the following year, the director of the MESC became a member of the Advisory Board of the National Undergraduate Program for Overseas Study of Arabic, probably the best undergraduate Arabic program ever devised. Supported by the Carnegie Foundation for about eight years and administered by Princeton, it consisted of one year of intensive instruction for eight students at the British Middle East Centre for Arab Studies in Shemlan, Lebanon. From the beginning, this program was dominated by students from Princeton and Portland State. In light of the general level of Arabic instruction in the United States at that time, it was not unusual for NUPOSA graduates who pursued advanced degrees in various fields of Middle Eastern studies to have a better command of Arabic than some of their professors in graduate school. This small group of alumni include Wheeler Thackston (Princeton) at Harvard, Rosalind Gwynne (Portland State) at Tennessee, and Fred Donner (Princeton) at the University of Chicago.

In 1964, the MESC pioneered in Arabic studies abroad on a large scale when it administered the first Summer Institute for Arabic Studies at the Center for Arabic Studies at the American University in Cairo. All 25 participants were undergraduates from Portland State. The following year there were three undergraduates (two from Portland State) and some 20 graduate students from throughout the United States. Again the MESC administered the program. This summer institute evolved into the current program at the Center for Arabic Studies Abroad at the American University in Cairo.

Noury played an important role in both the NUPOSA and Summer Institute in Cairo. Meanwhile, in 1962, he published *Arabic for Beginners*, one of the earliest manuals for introducing undergraduates to the Arabic writing system. In 1964, he introduced Arabic instruction at Wilson High School in Portland. In 1965 and 1966, he coordinated language instruction for Peace Corps projects in Turkey, Iran, Afghanistan, and Pakistan. At different times between 1965 and 1976, he directed the National Defense Education Act summer language institutes for secondary teachers of Arabic in the United States, participated in workshops on preparing Arabic text books at the University of Michigan and Columbia, did research on teaching Arabic to Arabs and non-Arabs in Egypt, Kuwait, Iraq, Jordan, and Saudi Arabia, and taught Arabic in summer programs at the universities of Utah, Washington, and elswhere. In 1980 he became director of the MESC.

In 1987, Noury retired as Professor Emeritus of Semitic Languages. During his almost three decades at Portland State, which became a university in 1969, he taught thousands of students. In fact, virtually every student who enrolled in the Middle Eastern program took one of his courses or seminars in Arabic, Ottoman Turkish, Islamic civilization or other topic. Many of these students later found careers in the United States Department of State or Department of Defense. Some now teach in various fields of Middle Eastern studies at such places as Princeton, Washington University, and Tulane University. Invariably, Noury's students would speak of him with affection, praising his warmth, patience, insightfullness, and tolerance. In a short speech on the occasion of the creation of a scholarship in Noury's name at Portland State, Farhat Ziadeh described him as a "secular-humanist, Eastern Orthodox, Congregational, Muslim." Altogether, Noury had a significant influence on a generation of students at Portland State who constituted a noticeable number of those Americans specializing in the Middle East. The present work testifies, to some degree, to that influence.

Gary Leiser, Director
Travis Air Museum
Travis AFB, California

INTRODUCTION*

Islamic civilization is rightly credited with making a number of advances in medicine, most notably in pharmacology, ophthalmology and the establishment of hospitals as genuine medical facilities.[1] From the beginning, Muslims took an avid interest in medicine and doctors were highly esteemed.[2] As the medical heritage of the lands conquered by Islam was absorbed and synthesized and the practice of medicine became more sophisticated, it was realized in many quarters that all recognized physicians should have a certain basic knowledge of medicine in order to protect the public from charlatans. Consequently, there was much discussion of a doctor's training and moral character. We know that as early as the third/ninth century examinations were sometimes given to determine a physician's qualifications.[3]

The oldest apparent Islamic medical examination to come to light bears the title *Imtiḥān al-alibbā' li-kāffat al-aṭibbā'* ["The Experts' Examination for All Physicians"]. It was prepared by 'Abd al-'Azīz al-Sulamī, the chief of medicine to the Ayyūbid sultan in Cairo between 596/1200 and 604/1208. It exists in three manuscripts found in Vienna, Bursa, and Cairo. The Bursa manuscript was copied by the personal physician of two Ottoman sultans in the tenth/sixteenth century, and the Vienna manuscript was in the possession of at least two chiefs of sultanal medicine of the Ottoman Empire in the thirteenth/nineteenth century. Thus, this work may have been used rather continuously in the heartland of the Islamic world from the medieval period until fairly recent times.

The Author

Our knowledge of the life of Muwaffaq al-Dīn 'Abd al-'Azīz ibn 'Abd al-Jabbār ibn Abī Muḥammad al-Sulamī al-Dimashqī is unfortunately very

* This introduction is a considerably revised version of al-Khaledy and Leiser's article "Bilinen en eski islam hekimlik sınavı" ["The Oldest Known Islamic Medical Examination"], *Hacettepe Üniversitesi Edebiyat Fakültesi Dergisi*, 5 (1987), pp. 166–84.

1 On the origin of Islamic hospitals, see Michael Dols, "The Origins of the Islamic Hospital: Myth and Reality," *BHM* 61 (1987), pp. 367–90.

2 See Franz Rosenthal, "The Physician in Medieval Muslim Society," *BHM* 52 (1978), pp. 475–91.

3 Gary Leiser, "Medical Education in Islamic Lands from the Seventh to the Fourteenth Century," *JHMS* 38 (1983), pp. 67–68.

sketchy. For the most part, what we know of him comes only indirectly from the material that we possess describing his family and associates. They were powerful and influential and therefore reflected his important status. As a result, the account that follows essentially provides the context of al-Sulamī's social world.

Our author was born in Syria, probably Damascus, around 550/1155 and died in Cairo in 604/1208. He was a member of the Sulamī family, which took its name from the Arab tribe of Sulaym. A branch of this tribe left Arabia during the early years of Islam and settled in Syria near Ḥimṣ.[4]

Throughout most of the sixth/twelfth century, the Sulamī family was especially prominent in Damascus in the field of Shāfi'ī law (*fiqh*). When the Amīniyya Madrasa, reputedly the first Shāfi'ī college of law in Damascus, was built in 514/1120, its professorship went to Jamāl al-Islām 'Alī ibn al-Musallam al-Sulamī (d. 533/1139). He had been a close associate of the famous Muslim theologian al-Ghazzālī when the latter visited Damascus in 488/1095. Indeed, he even taught law to al-Ghazzālī's circle of students in the Umayyad Mosque, next to which the Amīniyya was later built. 'Alī passed his professorship on to his son Abū Bakr Muḥammad (d. 564/1169), who was also the preacher of the Friday sermon (*khaṭīb*) and a professor of law in the Umayyad Mosque and a substitute for one of the chief judges of Damascus. Abū Bakr Muḥammad, in turn, passed his college professorship on to his son Sharaf al-Dīn 'Alī (d. 602/1206). 'Alī had previously taught tradition (*ḥadīth*) in Baghdad and Fusṭāṭ before succeeding his father.[5]

Although a *madrasa* traditionally had only one professorship that was, in theory, held for life, the length of tenure often depended on political,

---

4 Al-Sam'ānī, *Kitāb al-Ansāb*, ed. D.S. Margoliouth (Leiden: E.J. Brill, 1912), p. 303. The early history of the Sulamīs as a tribe has been described by Michael Lecker, *The Banū Sulaym: a Contribution to the Study of Early Islam* (Jerusalem: Magnes Press, 1989).

5 On the nature of the *madrasa*, see the works of George Makdisi, especially his *Rise of Colleges: Institutions of Learning in Islam and the West* (Edinburgh: Edinburgh University Press, 1981), and *EI* ^{2}, *s.v.* "Madrasa" (J. Pedersen/[G. Makdisi]). On the Amīniyya and its professors, see al-Nu'aymī, *al-Dāris fī ta'rīkh al-madāris*, ed. Ja'far al-Ḥasanī (Damascus: Maṭba'at al-Sharqī, 1367–70/1948–51), I, 177–205, index; Nikita Elisséeff, *Nūr ad-Dīn: un grand prince musulman de Syrie au temps des croisades (511–569 H/1118–1174)* (Damascus: Institut Français, 1967), III, 920. Ibn Shaddād ('Izz al-Dīn), *al-A'lāq al-khaṭīra*, Damascus section, ed. Sāmī al-Dahhān (Damascus: Institut Français, 1956), pp. 231–32, gives a somewhat different list of professors, which al-Nu'aymī believes is incorrect. Al-Subkī tends to support al-Nu'aymī, *Ṭabaqāt al-shāfi'iyya al-kubrā*, ed. Maḥmūd Muḥammad al-Ṭanāḥī and 'Abd al-Fattāḥ Muḥammad al-Ḥilū (Cairo: 'Īsā al-Ḥalabī, 1383–96/1964–76), cf. VII, 235–37, on Jamāl al-Islām, and VIII, 298, on Sharaf al-Dīn.

religious, or even personal considerations. Sometime after becoming the professor of the Amīniyya, Sharaf al-Dīn was expelled from Damascus and moved to Ḥimṣ, where he spent the rest of his life. This expulsion may have taken place when Quṭb al-Dīn Mas'ūd ibn Muḥammad al-Nīshābūrī al-Turaythīthī (d. 578/1183) became the professor of our *madrasa* in 568/1172–73. He was highly respected by the ruler of Syria, Nūr al-Dīn (d. 569/1174), and was the leading Shāfi'ī scholar of his time in Damascus. It is possible that the Sulamī family fell from favor under Nūr al-Dīn. The new master of Damascus did much to bring that city's religious leaders and intelligentsia into line with his particular policies towards both the Crusaders and other Muslim states.[6] Some no doubt would not conform. In any case, Quṭb al-Dīn was followed by Ḍiyā' al-Dīn 'Alī ibn 'Aqīl al-Dimashqī (d. 601/1205), who was succeeded by Ṣā'in al-Dīn 'Abd al-Wāḥid ibn Ismā'īl al-Dimyāṭī (d. 613/1216). The next two professors were Taqī l-Dīn 'Īsā ibn Yūsuf ibn Aḥmad al-'Irāqī (d. 601/1205–1206), who was involved in a scandal and committed suicide, and Jamāl al-Dīn Yūnus ibn Badrān al-Miṣrī (d. 623/1226), who was a chief judge and treasurer of Damascus and held other important posts.

Clearly, the Sulamī family lost control of the Amīniyya college in the second half of the sixth/twelfth century, and its professorship appears to have been caught up in Damascene politics. It was during this time that 'Abd al-'Azīz al-Sulamī began, and then abandoned, a career as a Shāfi'ī jurist. His early education was devoted to studying Shāfi'ī law in the Amīniyya, probably under Sharaf al-Dīn.[7] If the latter's departure for Ḥimṣ is an indication that the Sulamī family was out of favor while Nūr al-Dīn was in power, it was perhaps then that al-Sulamī found it expedient to specialize in medicine.

Whatever the circumstances, he excelled in this subject and had as a teacher the most outstanding physician of that period in Syria, Muwaf-

---

[6] On Nūr al-Dīn's policies, see Elisséeff, *Nūr ad-Dīn*, III, 750–79.

[7] The primary source for al-Sulamī's life is Ibn Abī Uṣaybi'a's *'Uyūn al-anbā' fī ṭabaqāt al-aṭibbā'* (Beirut: Dār Maktabat al-Ḥayāt, 1965), p. 671. Al-Ṣafadī's information comes from Ibn Abī Uṣaybi'a, *al-Wāfī bi-l-wafayāt*, ed. Hellmut Ritter *et al.* (Istanbul: Staatsdruckerei, 1931–proceeding), XVIII, 515, as does Carl Brockelmann's, *GAL S*, I, 894. Samira Jadon's statement that al-Sulamī taught theology in the Amīniyya is not supported by any evidence; see her "The Physicians of Syria during the Reign of Ṣalāḥ al-Dīn 570–589 A.H./1174–1193 A.D.," *JHMAS* 25 (1970), 338. Al-Sulamī is mentioned in passing in Anne-Marie Eddé, "Les médecins dans la société syrienne du VIIe/XIIIe siècle," *Annales Islamologiques* 29 (1995), 99. Ramazan Şeşen gives Ibn Abī Uṣaybi'a's account of him, "Eyyūbiler devrinde tip eğitimi" ["Medical Education in the Ayyūbid Period"], *İslâm Tetkikleri Dergisi*, 9 (1995), p. 231.

faq al-Dīn As'ad ibn Ilyās ibn al-Maṭrān (d. 587/1191). Born in Damascus, he spent virtually his entire life in his native city. After Saladin seized it in 571/1176 from Nūr al-Dīn's son and brought it under Ayyūbid control, Ibn al-Maṭrān became possibly the most important private doctor of the new ruler. He went with the sultan on campaign, treated his leading commanders (*amīrs*), and was apparently given the authority to oversee the promotions and fees of the physicians of Syria, whom he completely dominated. He was so greatly respected by Saladin, and his authority so increased, that he was almost regarded as a vizier. In addition, when Ibn al-Maṭrān converted to Islam from Christianity, the sultan gave him one of his concubines for a wife, a woman who had had considerable influence in his household.[8]

Another doctor and close friend of al-Sulamī was Muhadhdhab al-Dīn ibn al-Ḥājib (d. *ca.* 591/1195), who had been an engineer before practicing medicine. In fact, he used to maintain the clocks (*khadama fī l-sā'āt*) at the Umayyad Mosque. Because both men were interested in science and mathematics, they set out at one time for Mosul hoping to study under Sharaf al-Dīn al-Muẓaffar ibn Muḥammad al-Ṭūsī[9] (d. *ca.* 610/1213–14), the inventor of the "linear astrolabe," who was reportedly in that city. Unfortunately, he had left before they arrived. As a physician, Muhadhdhab al-Dīn later joined the service of Saladin's nephew, Taqī l-Dīn 'Umar ibn Shāhinshāh (d. 587/1191) in Ḥamāh. When Taqī l-Dīn died, he joined that of Saladin. After the latter's death he returned to Ḥamāh, where he himself passed away.[10]

Upon completing his medical studies, al-Sulamī practiced medicine in one of the greatest hospitals of the medieval Islamic world, the *bīmāristān* built by Nūr al-Dīn in Damascus.[11] It was here too that Ibn al-Maṭrān and Muhadhdhab al-Dīn had practiced. Apart from this, our doctor also gave public lectures on medicine for aspiring physicians. Although he certainly taught many students, the name of only one has come to light, Rashīd al-Dīn Abū l-Manṣūr ibn Abī l-Faḍl al-Ṣūrī (d. 639/1242), who also studied medicine from the well-known 'Abd al-Laṭīf al-Baghdādī (d. 629/1231–32). The latter made several trips to Damascus, the last in 604/1207–1208, and was a teacher of the fa-

[8] Ibn Abī Uṣaybi'a, *'Uyūn*, pp. 651–59; *GAL S*, I, 892; Manfred Ullmann, *Die Medizin im Islam* (Leiden and Köln: E.J. Brill, 1970), pp. 165–66, 191.

[9] Ibn Khallikān, *Wafayāt al-a'yān*, ed. Iḥsān 'Abbās (Beirut: Dār al-Thaqāfa, 1968–72), V, 314; VI, 52–53; *GAL*, I, 472, and *S*, I, 858; and *EI* [2], *s.v.* "Asṭurlāb" (W. Hartner), p. 727.

[10] Ibn Abī Uṣaybi'a, *'Uyūn*, pp. 659–60.

[11] *EI* [2], *s.v.* "Bīmāristān" (D.M. Dunlop *et al.*); Elisséeff, *Nūr ad-Dīn*, III, 838–43.

mous biographer of physicians Ibn Abī Uṣaybiʿa (d. 668/1270). Rashīd al-Dīn specialized in pharmacology and, beginning in 612/1215–16, served three successive Ayyūbid rulers of Damascus, al-ʿĀdil (r. 592–615/1196–1218), his son al-Muʿaẓẓam ʿĪsā (r. 615–24/1218–27), and his son al-Nāṣir Dāʾūd (r. 624–26/1227–29). The last appointed him "chief of medicine" (*raʾīs al-ṭibb*) in Damascus.[12]

Al-Sulamī undoubtedly helped bring Rashīd al-Dīn to al-ʿĀdil's attention, for he spent the last part of his life in that ruler's service. Al-Sulamī may have joined al-ʿĀdil when he captured Damascus in 592/1196 during the struggle for the Ayyūbid realm in the aftermath of Saladin's death. Al-ʿĀdil, who was one of Saladin's brothers, succeeded in gaining control of Egypt in 596/1200 and was proclaimed sultan of that country and Syria. Al-Sulamī was with him in Egypt. He was admired by the sultan and acquired a high position and much wealth.

That position must have been none other than chief of medicine in Egypt. This is clearly implied in an anecdote told about how the Damascene Muhadhdhab al-Dīn ʿAbd al-Raḥīm ibn ʿAlī al-Dakhwār (d. 628/1230) came to obtain that post. According to Ibn Abī Uṣaybiʿa:

> In the month of Shawwāl of the year 604 (April–May 1208), al-Malik al-ʿĀdil said to al-Ṣāḥib ibn Shukr (his vizier): "We need another physician to assist Muwaffaq al-Dīn ʿAbd al-ʿAzīz (al-Sulamī) with regard to serving the army and treating their illnesses. ʿAbd al-ʿAzīz can't keep up with all of this. Find someone like him!"

Al-Ṣāḥib recommended Muhadhdhab al-Dīn for the job and offered him a salary of 30 *dīnār*s a month. Muhadhdhab al-Dīn turned him down, however, saying: "My lord the physician Muwaffaq al-Dīn ʿAbd al-ʿAzīz receives 100 *dīnār*s and an equivalent amount of other income every month. I know my ability in this field and I will not take less!"[13] A month later, on Friday 20 Dhū l-Qaʿda/7 June, al-Sulamī suddenly died from a severe case of colitis, and Muhadhdhab al-Dīn took his place. He became *raʾīs al-ṭibb* and his responsibilities also included Syria, which was probably true for al-Sulamī.

Internal evidence from the *Imtiḥān* tends to confirm that al-Sulamī was chief of medicine (fol. 4b). Here we find that our doctor held an "of-

---

[12] Ibn Abī Uṣaybiʿa, *ʿUyūn*, pp. 699–703; Ullmann, *Medizin*, pp. 278–80. On the chief of medicine, see Leiser, "Medical Education," 71–73.

[13] Ibn Abī Uṣaybiʿa, *ʿUyūn*, p. 729; Ullmann, *Medizin*, p. 172. Al-Sulamī's salary was very handsome, see *EI*^{2}, *s.v.* "Dīnār" (G.C. Miles), and the relevant chapter on the cost of living in Eliyahu Ashtor, *Histoire des prix et des salaires dans l'orient médiéval* (Paris: Centre national de la recherche scientifique, 1969).

fice" (*wilāya*) and that al-Ṣāḥib had appointed him (*wallāhu*). The Arabic noun and verb used here were commonly used for appointments to official positions, although in this case the title of the post is not given. Furthermore, Ibn Abī Uṣaybiʿa tells us that Jamāl al-Dīn ʿUthmān ibn Hibat Allāh al-Qaysī (d. after 615/1218), known as Ibn Abī l-Ḥawāfir, was appointed the chief of medicine of Egypt by al-Malik al-ʿAzīz, al-ʿĀdil's nephew, who ruled that country from 589/1193 until his death in 595/1198.[14] Ibn Abī l-Ḥawāfir lost his job when al-ʿAzīz died. After Muhadhdhab al-Dīn, the next *ra'īs al-ṭibb* known in Egypt was the judge Nafīs al-Dīn Hibat Allāh ibn Ṣadaqa (d. 636/1238–39), who was appointed to that post by al-ʿĀdil's son and successor in Egypt, al-Malik al-Kāmil (d. 635/1238).[15] Therefore, al-Sulamī would fill the gap from at least 596/1200 to 604/1208 under al-ʿĀdil in the series of chiefs of medicine.

It is worthy of note that al-Sulamī dedicated his *Imtiḥān* to the vizier al-Ṣāḥib Ṣafī l-Dīn ʿAbd Allāh ibn ʿAlī ibn Shukr (d. 622/1225), and not to al-ʿĀdil, who is nowhere mentioned (fols. 2a, 5a). In fact, he praises al-Ṣāḥib in such high terms that one would think he was the sultan and not the vizier. But this may simply be because al-Ṣāḥib appointed him to his position.

As we shall see, the *Imtiḥān* was a fairly comprehensive "examination" which could be used to maintain certain medical standards in the Ayyūbid empire. Al-Sulamī lauds al-Ṣāḥib for his efforts to regulate and improve the practice of medicine (fol. 4b). It is possible that al-Ṣāḥib encouraged him to write the *Imtiḥān*, hence the dedication, although Ibn Abī Uṣaybiʿa makes no reference to any attempt by al-Ṣāḥib to improve medical standards under al-ʿĀdil. He only says that after Muhadhdhab al-Dīn became *ra'īs al-ṭibb*, al-ʿĀdil charged him with inspecting the practices of ophthalmologists and issuing them permits. This took place sometime before 614/1217–18.[16] Credit is given to the sultan, not to the vizier. And in 609/1212–13, al-Ṣāḥib was exiled from Egypt.

Virtually every account that we possess of the life of al-Ṣāḥib is hostile to him. He is described as an unsympathetic character in no uncertain terms, this despite the respect the religious classes had for him, his public works, and his construction of the only exclusively Mālikī *madrasa* in Cairo during the Ayyūbid period. Instead, we are told how he seized the wealth of leading government servants, confiscated the property of

---

[14] Ibn Abī Uṣaybiʿa, *ʿUyūn*, pp. 584–85.
[15] *Ibid.*, p. 586.
[16] *Ibid.*, p. 731.

leading families, and forced a number of judges to flee the country. The ruling circle, including al-ʿĀdil, eventually became exasperated with him and he was expelled from Egypt. Many anecdotes were told of his diabolical nature. For example, he was once stricken by such a severe case of dysentery that his doctors gave up hope for his recovery. While groaning in agony, he sent for ten shaykhs whom he had imprisoned. These men were then tortured in his presence. Their cries mixed with his, and he thus found company in their discomfort. This experience apparently provided the tonic he needed, for the next day he regained his health. In spite of the flaws in his character, he did fill the treasury and al-Kāmil later found it necessary to recall him to the vizierate.[17]

It is very likely that our sources have exaggerated the negative aspects of al-Ṣāḥib's vizierate. At least judging from al-Sulamī, he may well have been responsible for improving the state of the medical arts in the Ayyūbid Empire—perhaps as a result of his experience with dysentery—not to mention his public works and the like. It is certain that the *Imtiḥān* was written between 596/1200, when al-ʿĀdil became sultan of Egypt and al-Ṣāḥib became vizier, and 604/1208, when al-Sulamī died. By appointing al-Sulamī chief of medicine as well as finding his successor, Muhadhdhab al-Dīn, and encouraging him to write the *Imtiḥān*, as the text suggests, al-Ṣāḥib clearly had an interest in this aspect of the public welfare.[18]

As for al-Sulamī, we have few other details. In a few places in the *Imtiḥān* (fols. 24a–b), we learn that he was an observer of nature and experimented with *materia medica* (generally defined today as pharmacology). Ibn Abī Uṣaybiʿa reports that he was a very honorable man, generous, and kind. He would examine and treat the poor without a fee and pay for their drugs and dietary needs. He was pious, cheerful,

---

17 For the life of al-Ṣāḥib ibn Shukr, see Leiser, "The Restoration of Sunnism in Egypt: Madrasas and Mudarrisūn 495–647/1101–1249," Ph.D. dissertation, University of Pennsylvania 1976, pp. 318–21, 599; Hans L. Gottschalk, *al-Malik al-Kāmil von Egypten und seine Zeit* (Wiesbaden: Otto Harrassowitz, 1958), index; and Claude Cahen, "ʿAbdallaṭīf al-Baghdādī, portraitiste et historien de son temps," *BEO* 23 (1970), pp. 114–15.

18 It is worthy of note that a contemporary and, at least for a while, fellow countryman of al-Sulamī, the great Jewish physician and philosopher Moses Maimonides (534–601/1139–1204), wrote a work entitled *Treatise on Poisons and Their Antidotes* at the request of al-Qāḍī al-Fāḍil (d. 596/1200), Saladin's chief counselor and director of his chancellery. In this treatise, prepared in 595/1198, Maimonides praised al-Fāḍil for his concern for public welfare by ordering Egyptian physicians to store up supplies of certain important antidotes; English trans. Suessman Muntner (Philadelphia and Montreal: Lippincott, 1966), pp. 2–3.

and well liked by everyone.[19] When he died, the poet Ibn ʿUnayn (d. 630/1233), known more for ridiculing his subjects than praising them, was moved to say: "A unique man, just as no one follows the *khaṭīb*, there is no doctor after ʿAbd al-ʿAzīz."[20] Al-Sulamī passed away in Damascus and was buried on nearby Mt. Qāsyūn.

Finally, we should add that the author's son, Saʿd al-Dīn Ibrāhīm, became a famous physician in his own right. Born in Damascus in 583/1187, he devoted himself to the study of law, as his father had done, and became very prominent in that field. He subsequently took up medicine and practiced it in Nūr al-Dīn's hospital. Afterwards, he entered the service of another of al-ʿĀdil's sons, al-Ashraf Mūsā, who ruled Mayyāfāriqīn and Jabal Sinjar from 607/1210 to 617/1220 and in 626/1229 took over Damascus from his nephew al-Nāṣir Dā'ūd. Ibrāhīm seems to have been with him for most of this time, and in Damascus al-Ashraf appointed him chief of medicine. Ibrāhīm was, of course, a Shāfiʿī, and it is curious that, during al-Ashraf's reign in Damascus, he was placed in charge of the construction of the Jawziyya Ḥanbalī College near the Umayyad Mosque. This *madrasa* was built at the request of the ʿAbbāsid caliph al-Mustanṣir (r. 623–40/1226–42). When his overlord died in 635/1237, al-Kāmil confirmed him in his post of *ra'īs al-ṭibb*. Ibrāhīm remained in Damascus practicing and teaching medicine until he died in 644/1246.[21]

The Text

As we have seen, the *Imtiḥān al-alibbā' li-kāffat al-aṭibbā'* ["The Experts' Examination for All Physicians"] was written by al-Sulamī between 596/1200 and 604/1208 while he was the Ayyūbid chief of medicine in Cairo. In the introduction, he dedicates it to the vizier al-Ṣāḥib ibn Shukr, justifies the composition of medical books, praises the vizier for improving medical practice in the realm, and lastly states why he composed this work.

As noted above, the dedication is exceedingly laudatory and seems to place al-Ṣāḥib above the sultan. With regard to the justification, it was common for Muslim authors who wrote about subjects other than

---

19 Ibn Abī Uṣaybiʿa, *ʿUyūn*, p. 671.

20 Abū Shāma, *Dhayl ʿalā l-Rawḍatayn*, pub. under the title *Tarājim rijāl al-qarnayn al-sādis wa-l-sābiʿ* (Cairo: ʿIzzat al-ʿAṭṭār al-Ḥusaynī, 1366/1947), p. 63.

21 Ibn Abī Uṣaybiʿa, *ʿUyūn*, pp. 671–72; Ibn Wāṣil, *Mufarrij al-kurūb*, ed. Jamāl al-Dīn al-Shayyāl *et al.* (Cairo: Fouad I University Press, 1953–proceeding), V, 137, 220–21; al-Ṣafadī, *al-Wāfī*, VI, 48. On the Jawziyya Madrasa, see al-Nuʿaymī, *al-Dāris*, II, 29–63; Ibn Shaddād, *al-Aʿlāq*, pp. 256–57.

the religious sciences to preface their works with a description of their importance. This was done until fairly modern times. Religion was considered the most important scholarly subject, thus deserving the most attention. Writers on non-religions topics, therefore, frequently found it necessary to begin their works with an apologia, an explanation of how their treatises were related, if not essential, to the religious sciences.[22] Al-Sulamī was no exception and he tells us of the vital role ascribed to medicine by such men as the Prophet Muḥammad himself and the great legal scholar al-Shāfiʿī. Next, the author praises the vizier for his actions in weeding out incompetent physicians. It is clearly implied that the vizier's efforts in this respect led al-Sulamī to compose the *Imtiḥān*, if he were not specifically requested to do so. We are then told that the book was written "so that one can ascertain with it the knowledge of someone who claims to know this art and how much he understands, and reveal the quality of his knowledge and practice" (fol. 5a).

Al-Sulamī divided his work into ten chapters, each containing twenty questions on a particular branch of medicine. In addition, he provided an answer for each question and almost always cited a source for it. When the source of an answer is not given, it can reasonably be assumed to be found in one of the books cited in that chapter. Moreover, the answers are provided, says the author, so that an examiner would have an authoritative source should a respondent give a different answer. It would appear, therefore, that this examination could be given by someone with little or no medical training.[23] It should be mentioned, how-

---

[22] See Franz Rosenthal, "The Defense of Medicine in the Medieval Muslim World," *BHM* 43 (1969), pp. 522–25.

[23] Here, of course, that renowned figure, the supervisor of moral behavior and the marketplace, the *muḥtasib*, comes to mind. On his role as a medical inspector, see Leiser, "Medical Education," 72; especially Michael W. Dols, *Medieval Islamic Medicine: Ibn Riḍwān's Treatise "On the Prevention of Bodily Ills in Egypt"* (Berkeley: University of California Press, 1984), p. 33 n. 170, and p. 34, n. 172; and Lawrence I. Conrad, "Usāma ibn Munqidh and Other Witnesses to Frankish and Islamic Medicine in the Era of the Crusades," in Efraim Lev, ed., *Medicine in Jerusalem through the Ages* (Tel Aviv: Bar Elan University Press, 1998), pp. 23–24. For a discussion of the customary view of the state control of medicine in medieval Muslim society, see Ghada Karmi, "State Control of the Physicians in the Middle Ages: An Islamic Model," in A.W. Russell, ed., *The Town and State Physician in Europe from the Middle Ages to the Enlightenment* (Wolfenbüttel: Herzog August Bibliothek, 1981), pp. 63–84; and cf. Dols, *Medieval Islamic Medicine*, pp. 32–36. H.D. Isaacs has published an interesting medical certificate from the Cairo Geniza. Dated 1262, it was issued by two men who were either doctors or representatives of the government and was a kind of official notice that a certain person had leprosy, "A Medieval Arab Medical Certificate," *Medical History* 35 (1991), 250–57, cf. Gary Leiser and Michael Dols, "Evliyā Chelebi's Description of Medicine in Seventeenth-Century

ever, that to the extent that the answers can be compared to the sources cited, most of them are clearly paraphrases or summaries of passages from these sources. The lack of context for such answers would have bewildered a non-specialist. In fact, the lack of context sometimes makes it difficult to determine the antecedents of many pronouns and even the subject of many sentences in the answers. Furthermore, in a field like pharmacology, in which there were a great many unfamiliar names of plants, a non-specialist could easily misread various names. This is obvious from the discrepancies between the present text and corresponding passages in Ibn Wāfid, who is cited on many drugs.

The questions and answers in the *Imtiḥān* were derived from the material found in certain medical texts that were well-known and readily available. Altogether they numbered about 25 books by some seventeen writers. Some chapters of the examination depend primarily on one or two authorities and others on many:

Chapter I (the pulse): mainly Galen and Ibn Sīnā
Chapter II (urine): Isḥāq ibn Sulaymān al-Isrā'īlī
Chapter III (fevers and crises): Galen
Chapter IV (symptoms): 'Alī ibn al-'Abbās al-Majūsī
Chapter V (simple drugs): Ibn Wāfid
Chapter VI (treatment): Ibn Sīnā
Chapter VII (the eye): 'Alī ibn 'Īsā
Chapter VIII (surgery): many writers
Chapter IX (bonesetting): Ibn Sīnā and al-Majūsī
Chapter X (fundamentals): many writers

Of the 200 questions, Ibn Sīnā answers at least 58; al-Majūsī at least 41; and Galen at least 34, for a total of 133. Many books by Galen are cited, but for Ibn Sīnā chiefly his *al-Qānūn* and for al-Majūsī only his *al-Malakī*. In three cases, I:7, III:16, VIII:1, and VIII:13 (?), two somewhat different answers are given, and in another, V:4, the author himself criticizes part of the answer and furnishes his own clarification.

The *Imtiḥān* raises several interesting questions. First, is it really an "examination"? Al-Sulamī expressly states that this is the case, yet his work clearly falls into a genre of Islamic writings generally known as "question and answer" literature. The question and answer format was used in many fields and became a fairly common means of disputing various philosophical or cosmological issues. In medicine, the archetypical example of this format was Ḥunayn ibn Isḥāq's (d. 260/873) *Masā'il fī*

Egypt," pt. 2, *Sudhoffs Archiv* 72 (1988), 53.

l-ṭibb li-l-muta'allimīn.[24] In this field, the question and answer pattern has been described as serving "an exclusively didactic purpose, namely the transmission of specific knowledge."[25] But how so? As will be seen from the *Imtiḥān*, it presupposes a thorough understanding of the theory and practice of Galenic medicine. An aspiring physician could acquire this understanding in two basic ways, either by studying the relevant texts on his own or with a teacher. If a student were self-taught, the *Imtiḥān* would be pointless as a didactic device because he could obviously consult the full original texts whenever he wished. Consequently, a work like the *Imtiḥān* would only have been of didactic value between a teacher and student. In other words, a teacher could have used it as a kind of "crib book" or crude syllabus to ensure that his students had mastered a certain body of material. It was not a "catechism" in the sense of a summary of fundamental information. Instead it provided a framework for, and guide to, specific information. It was, therefore, not a formal "examination" that was given to students after they had completed their studies, nor was it given to certify practicing physicians. There is internal evidence in the *Imtiḥān* confirming that it was used simply as a teaching tool. Al-Sulamī answers question V.4, on simple drugs, by citing an authoritative source at some length and then adds his own equally lengthy criticism of that source. And in the answer to question VIII.4, on what a surgeon should be asked, the author adds to the authoritative source a comment on a marginal note that he found in a copy of that source. If the *Imtiḥān* had been a formal "examination," only al-Sulamī's students might have known this. When the author speaks of having written this work "so that one can ascertain with it the knowledge of someone who claims to know this art and how much he understands, and reveal the quality of his knowledge and practice," he must be referring only to his or other students. And when he states that he provided answers to questions so that an examiner would have an authoritative source if the respondent gave a different answer, the "examiner" could only have been himself or another teacher. In this context, it could be argued that the *Imtiḥān* was, at best, an "informal" examination, as well a crib book, because it helped ensure that al-Sulamī's students had covered the material.

Second, how much of the *Imtiḥān* was one expected to master? The

---

[24] English trans. by Paul Ghalioungui as *Questions on Medicine for Scholars* (Cairo: Al-Ahram Center for Scientific Translations, 1980). As will be seen, some of al-Sulamī's questions parallel those of Ḥunayn.

[25] *EI*^{2}, *s.v.* "Masā'il wa-adjwiba" (H. Daiber), p. 637.

answer is not clear. Al-Sulamī implies in his introduction that general practitioners should have a knowledge of all ten fields in the work. On the other hand, the titles of some chapters, such as IX: "On What the Bonesetter Should be Asked," certainly suggest that one could master part of it according to his speciality.[26] This raises a related question, how did one master a field? Did he simply need a general knowledge of the authoritative works in that field so that he could refer to them as cases arose, or did he need to memorize all or parts of those works? In an important article on the role of memorization in traditional Islamic education, Dale Eickelman points out how, with respect to the religious sciences, knowledge remained constant over time and that mastery of this knowledge depended on which texts one had memorized, beginning with the Qur'ān. Years were devoted to this endeavor. "As for secular knowledge," he states, "... it includes knowledge related to commerce and crafts, including music and oral poetry. These have significant parallels in form with the religious sciences and are also presumed to be contained by fixed, memorizable truths."[27] It seems to me, however, that such a presumption would be incautious, at least with respect to such secular knowledge as astronomy, mathematics, and medicine. Certainly some material in these fields was memorized simply in the course of studying or practicing the profession, but it would be rash to expect, much less require, more than that. Al-Sulamī's *Imtiḥān* is revealing in this regard. If we were to take it at face value as simply an examination, we would expect one who took it to have memorized as many as two dozen books, some of which ran to numerous volumes, depending on how many fields of medicine he was expected to have mastered. How else could he answer such questions as: "How many useful, hot, and dry medicines in the third degree are there? How many are hot and moist, cold and dry, and cold and moist (V:20)?" The response was to enumerate 88 specific substances mentioned by Ibn Wāfid. Or: "How many uses are there for oxymel (VI:10)?" The answer was to list 88 uses recorded by Ibn al-Mudawwar. Or: "What is the 54th aphorism of the fourth treatise of Hippocrates' *al-Fuṣūl* and what is the meaning of it (X:14)?" Here the reply had to include a direct quotation. Can we have

---

26 Isḥāq ibn 'Alī al-Ruhāwī (fl. third/ninth cent.) states in his *Adab al-ṭabīb* that a physician should be examined according to his specialty; see Martin Levey, trans., *Medical Ethics of Medieval Islam with Special Reference to al-Ruhāwī's "Practical Ethics of the Physician"* (Philadelphia: American Philosophical Society, 1967), pp. 15, 81.

27 "The Art of Memory: Islamic Education and Its Social Reproduction," *Comparative Studies in Society and History* 20 (1978), 491.

expected a prospective physician to have memorized the work of any of these writers (the *materia medica* of Ibn Wāfid would be staggering) much less Ibn Sīnā's massive *al-Qānūn*? It would mock credulity.[28] Moreover, because so many answers to the "examination" are summaries or paraphrases of the works cited, it is obvious that memorization had its limits. Medicine, after all, was a practical craft, a professional way of earning one's living. It made no sense to spend years memorizing medical texts when one's remuneration depended on getting into the business as quickly as possible.[29] It sufficed to understand the contemporary theory of medicine, to be able to read, and to know which books to consult as needed. The *Imtiḥān*, as a didactic tool, perfectly suited this purpose.

Finally, how common were works like the *Imtiḥān* and what was their impact? Medical texts in the question and answer format were written from at least the time of Ḥunayn ibn Isḥāq (third/ninth century) to the time of al-Sulamī (seventh/thirteenth century) and remained in circulation, and presumably in use, until the thirteenth/nineteenth century, judging from the owners of al-Sulamī's work.[30] They all inculcated and strengthened the Galenic view of medicine, the professional and "scientific" medicine of the day. To the extent that they did so, they were a significant tool in the struggle against charlatanism, i.e., non-Galenic medicine. Galenic medicine, which required considerable study, "worked." Non-Galenic medicine did not and could have dan-

---

28 With respect to memorization, the physician Ibn Jumay', an Egyptian contemporary of al-Sulamī, states the following in his *al-Maqāla al-ṣalāḥiyya fī iḥyā' al-ṣinā'a al-ṣiḥḥiyya*, trans. Hartmut Fähndrich as *Treatise to Ṣalāḥ ad-Dīn on the Revival of the Art of Medicine* (Wiesbaden: Franz Steiner, 1983), p. 13: "This is also the case with all other arts similar to the art of medicine, that is to say, mastery of each art can only be attributed to some one—who is then deservedly credited with it—on the basis of two factors: first, the acquisition as actual memorized material of all the information this art encompasses; and second, the attainment of the capability to act on the basis of this information on particulars. Therefore, the learned have defined practical art as the potential to act on the basis of knowledge. It is impossible to attain this capability to act on the basis of the information of a particular art from the study of material in books written on that art, because books only contain general, common things. As regards particulars, that is to say characteristics of one single healthy or sick individual, books cannot contain them.... Rather, one attains this capability only through extensive practice, training, and [the development of] skillfulness, while practicing medicine, and through much perserverance in its particulars, after the practitioner had first attained a firm knowledge of the information pertaining to it expecially under the supervision of skilled teachers."

29 Also, unlike the Qur'ān, medical texts were not in rhymed prose. And there was no religious or spiritual merit in memorizing them.

30 For more examples, see Ullmann, *Medizin*, pp. 110, 166, 127, 209.

gerous consequences. By writing the *Imtiḥān*, al-Sulamī helped maintain standards, as they were understood at the time, and thus fulfilled his duties as chief of medicine in Cairo. In this capacity, he may even have required all teachers of medicine in the state to use his work. We do not know. It is noteworthy that the *Imtiḥān* mentions no need for clinical experience, which anyway was not necessary for learning Galenic medicine, nor does it refer to any license or certification that was given to anyone who mastered the material. Indeed, there is little evidence from any source that anything like a "board of medical examiners" was ever instituted.[31] Again judging from the *Imtiḥān*, it would appear that the responsibility for maintaining standards, namely, enforcing Galenism, rested primarily on individual teachers and the chiefs of medicine who supervised them. As long as Galenic medicine was taught, the public was safe.

We can, therefore, sum up the significance of the *Imtiḥān* in several ways. First, it sheds light on the position of the chief of medicine, revealing some of his responsibilities and how he could carry them out. Second, it gives us an insight into contemporary methods of teaching medicine. Third, it introduces us to contemporary medical standards, telling us what the major branches of medicine were and what the trained physician was expected to know about them. It reveals in particular what were regarded as the primary texts for each branch of medicine. We should emphasize that, by the beginning of the seventh/thirteenth century, classical Islamic civilization had reached its zenith.[32] Most of the great medical books had been written. Thus, al-

31 The *Livre des assises de la cour des bourgeois* ["Ordinances of the Court of Burgesses"] compiled between 1240 and 1244 in the Crusader-controlled city of Acre included a requirement that anyone, Muslim or Christian, who wished to practice medicine within that Frankish kingdom had to submit to an examination before the best physicians of the land. See Conrad, "Usāma ibn Munqidh," pp. 5, 22–24. There is somewhat more information on how a physician should be formally examined. This literature focuses on the kinds of questions to ask and the type of moral behavior and personality that should be sought. There is no evidence, however, that such examinations were systematically given. See Leiser, "Medical Education," pp. 68–70, to which add Albert Dietrich, *Medicinalia Arabica* (Göttingen: Vandenhoeck and Ruprecht, 1966), pp. 190–95; Ullmann, *Medizin*, pp. 223–26; Dols, *Medieval Islamic Medicine*, pp. 32–22; Fähndrich, *Treatise to Ṣalāḥ ad-Dīn*, pp. 28–35; Albert Z. Iskandar, *Galen: On Examinations by Which the Best Physicians are Recognized* (Berlin: Akademie-Verlag, 1988); Lawrence I. Conrad, "The Arab-Islamic Medical Tradition," in Conrad *et al.*, *The Western Medical Tradition, 800 BC to AD 1800* (Cambridge: Cambridge University Press, 1995), pp. 131–32.

32 See, e.g., S.D. Goitein, "The Four Faces of Islam," in his *Studies in Islamic History and Institutions* (Leiden: E.J. Brill, 1968), pp. 42–46, and the various articles in D.S. Richards, ed., *Islamic Civilization 950–1150* (Oxford: Cassirer, 1973).

Sulamī's work epitomized, to a great degree, the most advanced medical knowledge that this civilization produced.[33] Lastly, we might mention that it provides a brief glimpse of at least one book that has not survived, namely, Qusṭā ibn Lūqā's *Madkhal ilā 'ilm al-ṭibb*.

Galenic Medicine

Before describing the known manuscripts of the *Imtiḥān*, a few words are in order about Galenic medicine. As mentioned above, our text presumes a complete understanding of this theory of medicine. The answers to most of its questions are comprehensible only within this theoretical framework. Drawing from Aristotle, Hippocrates and other sources, Galen of Pergamum (d. *ca.* 216) created the final synthesis of the medical knowledge of antiquity. This synthesis became the medical standard in the Mediterranean world for thirteen centuries. In the Middle East, in fact, it remained the predominant medical system, regardless of religion, until the nineteenth century. It permeates almost all the works cited by al-Sulamī.

The essence of Galen's system was humoral pathology. He held that all things were composed of different combinations of four elements: earth, air, fire, and water, which embodied four primary and opposite fundamental qualities, hot, cold, wet and dry. Anything that was ingested was cooked by natural heat and transformed into different substances. Four humors or liquids resulted: blood, phlegm, black bile, and yellow bile. Balance among these humors created good health. Excess or defect of one humor or another gave rise to illness. Balance and various types of imbalance were categorized as different temperaments. Remedies for illnesses were sought in treatments thought to have an opposite effect. Thus if an illness were believed to result from imbalance toward cold and moist, it would be treated with drugs considered to be hot and dry. Other factors, such as sleep, emotional state, exercise, eating and drinking habits, evacuation and retention, and environment were also regarded as influential and were incorporated into the humoral system. Altogether this was a completely self-contained system which could answer virtually any question about one's health.

As for Galen's explanation of the physiological process, he asserted that it was controlled by the interaction of three basic faculties or forces: the natural, which were manifest in conception, growth, and nourish-

[33] For an excellent overview of the state of medical knowledge and practice in the medieval Muslim world, see Dols, *Medieval Islamic Medicine*, pp. 3–42. Dols' work is both an overview of this subject and a guide for students.

ment; the vital or animal, which were manifest in the heart and arteries; and the psychic, which determined thought, emotion, and voluntary movement. The natural originated in the liver and were distributed through the veins. The vital were created in the heart and were distributed through the arteries. And the psychic were found in the brain and were distributed through the nerves. Furthermore, each faculty had its own "pneuma" which, in conjunction with innate heat, broke down life-giving material and distributed it to different parts of the body.[34]

Manuscripts of the Arabic Text

As mentioned, there are three known manuscripts of the *Imtiḥān*. They are found in Vienna, Bursa, and Cairo. Because it was frequently copied and used as late as the thirteenth/nineteenth century, as can be seen from the dates of the physicians who owned the Vienna version, other copies may eventually come to light. Carl Brocklemann says a Hindustani translation was published in Dehli by M. Badr al-Dīn Khān Dahlawī in 1318/1900,[35] but we have not seen it.

All three of our manuscripts were copied long after the death of the author. The Bursa and Cairo manuscripts are clearly dated 1562 and 1683, respectively. The date of the Vienna manuscript is partly illegible, probably 1528 or 1626. It may thus be the earliest. It is the most complete and error free of the three copies. Each manuscript has some gaps, words, phrases, or errors unique to itself. In addition, the Bursa and Cairo manuscripts have many words, phrases, or errors in common which are not found in the Vienna manuscript. At the same time, all three manuscripts have a few gaps or oversights (some quirky) in common. For example, in VI:10, items number 17, 26, and 27 in the answer are missing from all three manuscripts. The same is true of item number six in the answer to X:20. And whereas in V:19, a question about the number of certain medicines, the answer given is "nine but he copied eight," after which ten are listed. These discrepancies in particular mean that our three manuscripts were descended from the same copy of the *Imtiḥān*, and one that bore a certain number of mistakes. They cannot be traced back to the original work. Furthermore, because of the special similarities between the Bursa and Cairo manuscripts, they must repre-

---

[34] For an introduction to Galenism with special reference to the Islamic world, see Ullmann, *Medizin*, pp. 56–64; Dols, *Medieval Islamic Medicine*, pp. 3–24; and Lawrence I. Conrad, *s.v.* "Medicine" in John Esposito, ed., *The Oxford Encyclopedia of the Modern Islamic World* (Oxford: Oxford University Press, 1995).

[35] *GAL S*, I, 894.

sent a stem from the ultimate common copy that is different from that of the Vienna manuscript.

The Vienna Manuscript (Mixt. 1408.1, fols. 1a–56a)[36]

This copy of our manuscript was purchased in Istanbul in 1933 and is the first of two works bound together in one volume. The second work is a commentary on Hippocrates (Mixt. 1408.2) by a different author and in a different hand. Between these two texts are a few poems in Persian, one by Ibn Sulṭān Shāh, and various religious notes. At the very end are a number of medical notes, partly in verse, and mostly in Persian. The manuscript is written on brownish, thick, glossy oriental paper, which in many places is soiled or deeply water-stained. It is 56 folios in length. Each page is 19.2 × 15 cm. and has 17 lines. The *naskh* script in which the manuscript is written is generally straight and clear, but virtually without diacritical points and very often without dots. Oversized lettering is used for part of the dedication and for the number of each chapter and question. Somewhat smaller letters are used for the word "answer" (*al-jawāb*) to each question. Red ink is used for each chapter title and for the word "answer." Apart from this, black ink is used throughout.

The copyist confused a few of the names of the *materia medica*, for most of these names are in languages other than Arabic, especially Persian.[37] In some multi-part answers, he sometimes accidently left out one or two items. There are also some words and a few phrases missing elsewhere. There are almost no corrections or marginal notes.

The beginning and ending of the text of this manuscript does not differ from the other two. There is a title page, however, on which are the names of many people who owned this particular copy at one time or another. Their names are as follows: Rūḥī, the professor (*al-mudarris*), Yūsuf ibn Muṣṭafā; Ḥannā, the physician (*al-ḥakīm*)....; Aḥmad ibn Ibrāhīm ibn Shihāb al-Islām, the doctor (*al-ṭabīb*); Muḥammad ibn Muṣṭafā; Ḥannā al-Ḥalabī, the doctor; Muṣṭafā Mas'ūd...., 1226 (1811); Muṣṭafā Bahjat, chief of sultanal medicine (*ra'īs al-aṭibbā'*

36 Helen Loebenstein, *Katalog der arabischen Handschriften der Österreichischen Nationalbibliothek* (Vienna: Hollinek in Komm., 1970), pp. 187, 283.

37 Admittedly, the identification of various drugs in lists of *materia medica* was a frequent problem for Arab physicians and pharmacologists, beginning with the Arabic translation of Dioscorides' famous book on this subject in the third/ninth century. See Albert Dietrich, "Islamic Sciences and the Medieval West: Pharmacology," in Khalil I. Semaan, ed., *Islam and the Medieval West* (Albany: State University of New York Press, 1980), pp. 50–63.

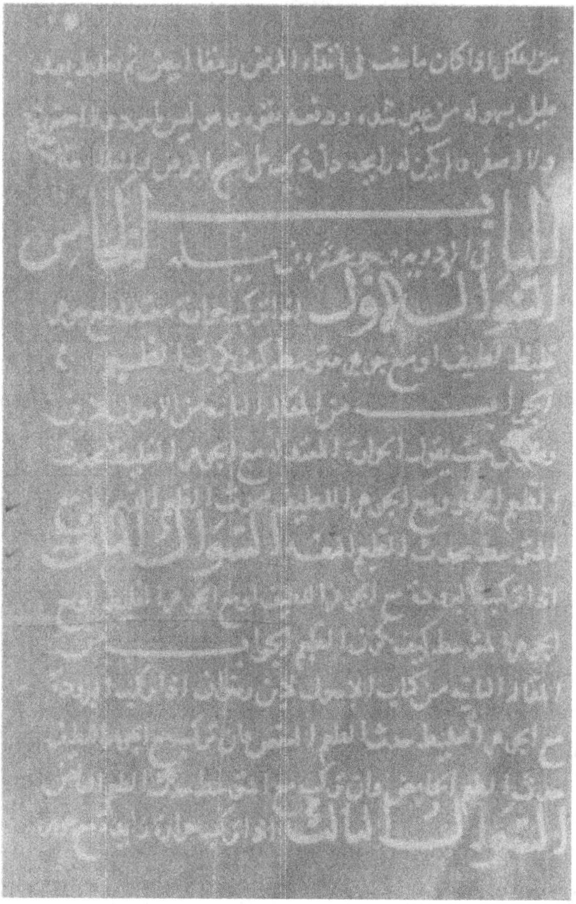

Figure 1: Vienna manuscript fol. 23a.

al-sulṭāniyya, 1221 (1806–1807); 'Abd al-Ḥaqq, chief of sultanal medicine, 1250 (1834–35); and Abū Naṣr Bahā' al-Dīn. There are three seals, two on the title page and one on fol. 2a. One of the first two bears the name al-Ḥājj Muṣṭafā, 1179 (1765–66). The others are illegible, but are also from the Ottoman period.

At the end of the manuscript is the following colophon: "This was finished on 14 Ramaḍān in the year 35 and was written by the slave Muḥammad ibn. . . al-Rūmī. . . ." The date of the colophon is probably 14 Ramaḍān, 935/22 May, 1528 or 1035/9 June, 1626. The copyist cannot be identified.

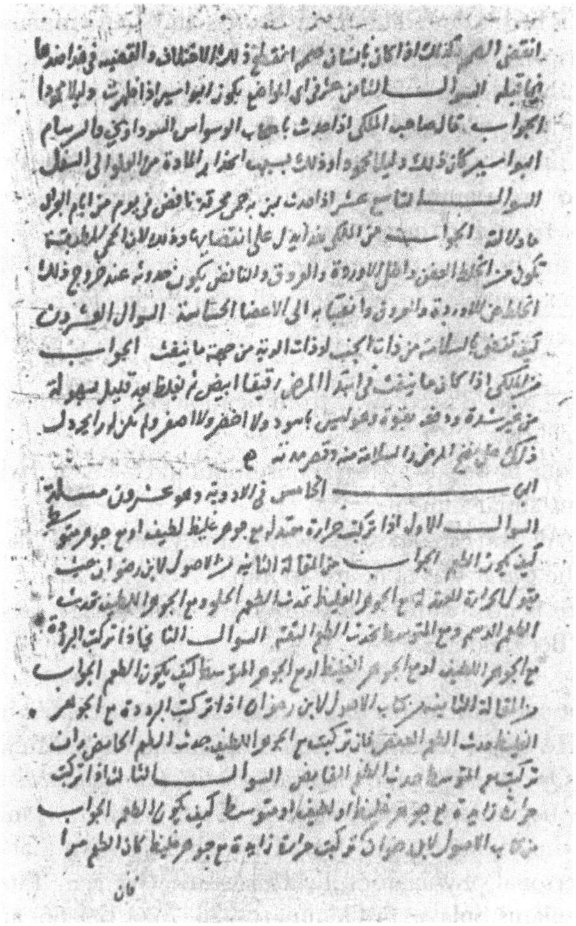

Figure 2: Bursa manuscript fol. 29a.

The Bursa Manuscript (Haraççı-oğlu 1120, fols. 19a–46b)[38]

This copy of the *Imtiḥān* is the second of six works on medicine bound together in one volume. Each work is by a different author: Galen, al-Sulamī, Abū l-Faraj ʿAlī ibn Hindū, al-Ghazzālī, Muḥammad ibn Qāsim al-Ḥarīrī, and al-Rāzī. All were copied by the same person. Our manuscript is written on glossy brown paper and is 27 folios in length. Each page is 20.8 x 15.1 cm. and has 22 small lines. It is written in black ink in a sloping (*taʿlīq*), hurried, *naskh* script, which is without diacritical

38 Dietrich, *Medicinalia*, pp. 190, 195–98.

points but is better dotted than the Vienna and Cairo manuscripts. The hurried script, however, makes it somewhat more difficult to read. Oversized, or rather, elongated letters are used to set off the beginning of each chapter and question, and to a certain extent for the word "answer." In multi-part answers, a straight line is drawn over the first word of each part. There are a number of corrections and marginal notes, although minor gaps remain in the text.

Before the body of the text begins one finds the following verses, which emphasize the role of God's will in providing for good health and suggest a certain fatalism:

> Hippocrates passed away from hemiplegia, Plato died from pleurisy,
> Aristotle passed away from consumption, Galen died with an intestinal ailment,
> Abū 'Alī (Ibn Sīnā) passed away from dysentery one day and the *Qānūn* was of no use to him,
> There is no treatment for any disease unless He says of it "Be!" and it is.[39]

As mentioned, the entire Bursa manuscript was copied by the same person. He was Muḥammad ibn Muḥammad ibn Muḥammad al-Qawṣūnī (Qaysūnizāde), the medical practitioner (*mutaṭabbib*).[40] Indeed, at the very beginning of this collection of works, al-Qawṣūnī states that it was he who copied them. Albert Dietrich has shown that our copyist was the personal physician of the *khān* of the Crimean Tatars and the Ottoman sultans Sulaymān Qānūnī (r. 926–74/1520–66) and Selim II (r. 974–82/1566–74). The date of his death is not known.[41]

At the end of our manuscript there is the following colophon:

> It was finished on 11 Rabīʿ I in the year 970 (8 November 1562). Praise be to God... Muḥammad ibn Muḥammad ibn Muḥammad al-Qawṣūnī wrote it. May God look kindly upon him and on all Muslims. May God

39 Cf. Qur'ān 16:40 and 36:82; trans. Arthur J. Arberry, *The Koran Interpreted* (New York: Macmillan, 1970), I, 290; II, 149.

40 On the distinction between a *ṭabīb* and *mutaṭabbib*, see Dols, *Medieval Islamic Medicine*, p. 28 n. 139.

41 *Medicinalia*, p. 190; also Ullmann, *Die Medizin*, pp. 180–81. It is worthy of note that the work by Galen that al-Qawṣūnī copied as part of this collective volume was Ḥunayn ibn Isḥāq's Arabic translation of his *De optimo medici cognoscendo*, in Arabic *Fī l-miḥna allatī yuʿrafu bihā afāḍil al-aṭibbā'*. This has been edited and translated by Albert Z. Iskandar as *Galen: On Examinations by Which the Best Physicians are Recognized*.

> bless our master Muḥammad, his family and all his companions. Praise be to God the Lord of the worlds....

At the beginning of this collection of manuscripts are three seals of ownership, and at the end there is an endowment seal that reads:

> This book, which was in his possession, was given as a pious endowment to the library attached to the new Naqshbandī *zāwiya* (corner of a mosque, lodge) in Bursa, to be studied as part of the education available in the mosque on condition that it not be removed from it, year 1163 (1749–50).[42]

The Cairo Manuscript (Dār al-Kutub, VI, 32 ṭibb)[43]

This copy of our text is the last of four works bound together in one volume entitled *al-Jawhar al-nafīs*. This title is simply part of the name of the first work, which is apparently a commentary on medicine, composed in 1093/1682. The second work is a medical text, the author of which died in 1005/1596–97, and the third is a treatise on palm reading, the author of which died in 606/1209–1210. Each work is in a different hand. Our manuscript is written on brownish paper and is 34 folios (67 pages) in length, although it is without folio or page numbers. Each page is 81.5 x 11 cm. and has 25 lines. It is written in black ink in *naskh* script that often has diacritical points and is fairly well dotted. Oversized letters are used for each chapter heading and slightly larger letters are used for each question number and the word "answer."

As the latest of our three manuscripts, this one has the most mistakes: elementary grammar errors, misspellings, and words that are switched around or missing. In fact, compared to the other manuscripts, not only phrases but whole sentences are sometimes missing. And a gap is left in the text for the last question and answer in the third chapter. There are a few corrections and no marginal notes.

At the end is the following colophon:

> This copy was finished on Monday the blessed on 6 Jumādā I, 1094 (3 May 1683)... by al-Faqīr Yūsuf ibn Muḥammad ibn Yūsuf al-Wakīl whose country is Malū (Mali?) and whose law school is Shāfiʿī. May God pardon him, his parents... his brothers and all Muslims.

---

42 The role of the Ṣūfī brotherhoods in the history of Islamic medicine has not been investigated. For one hint of it, see, for example, Leiser and Dols, "Evliyā Chelebi's Description of Medicine," pt. 2, p. 52.

43 *Fihrist al-kutub al-ʿarabiyya al-maḥfūẓa bi-l-kutubkhāna al-khidīwiyya al-miṣriyya* (Cairo, AH 1306–1309), VI, 32 no. 4300.

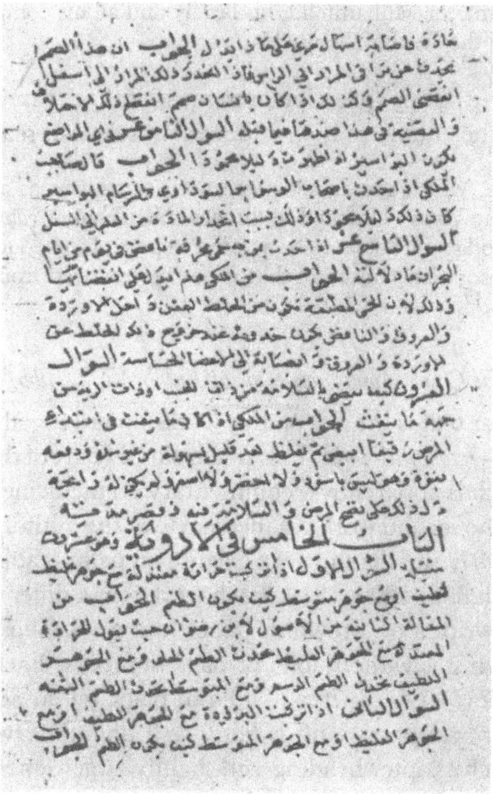

Figure 3: Cairo manuscript fol. 26a.

The Present Edition

Because the Vienna manuscript may have been the earliest of those in our possession and is the most complete and has the fewest errors, we have generally, but not exclusively, used it as the controlling version of the text. The folio numbers in the edition and translation correspond to those of the Vienna manuscript. These numbers are meant to facilitate the comparison of the edition with the translation. In those cases in which al-Sulamī's text can be checked against the sources he cites, such as Ibn Sīnā's *al-Qānūn*, these sources are used to control the text (although the 1294/1877 edition of *al-Qānūn* used here has flaws of its own). This can only be done, of course, with those sources that have been published. Moreover, it must be kept in mind that when al-Sulamī cites a source he may do so verbatim or only provide a paraphrase or summary.

Sometimes, in fact, he gives a "mixed" citation. Furthermore, because of the lack of context for much of the text, and the special knowledge required to understand it, we can be sure that most copyists had only a vague notion of what they were transcribing. Indeed, confusion in the manscripts with regard to the gender of certain words, the antecedents of many pronouns, and even the subject of some passages is clear evidence of this. Consequently, the "correct" reading in some cases may still be a bit problematic. All major differences among the manuscripts and the sources cited, if published, have been indicated in the notes to the edition. Differences in dotting are noted only if this could result in a different reading of a word. If the context clearly indicates how a word lacking dots should be read, the differences in dotting are not noted. The copyists very rarely put in a *hamza*. Instead, they indicated it by a *yā* or *kursī*, such as a *wāw* or *alif maqṣūra*. We have inserted all *hamza*s. Finally, all words enclosed in square brackets in the translation are implied in the text but are not actually there. All words enclosed in parentheses in the translation are explanations or clarifications.

THE EXPERTS' EXAMINATION FOR ALL PHYSICIANS

IN THE NAME OF GOD, THE COMPASSIONATE, THE MERCIFUL

[1b] Praise be to God who granted the benefits of reason, bestowed all other blessings, created man and taught him what he did not know, and made for him from animals, plants, and minerals that which will preserve his health, by His permission, and eliminate illness. God bless and grant salvation to our master Muḥammad, the Seal of the Prophets, and his family.

The light of science has shone and its wonders have become manifest after a period of obscurity. The spirits of its masters have become strong, and its seekers have high aspirations. The qualified are in high demand and enlightened men have come to power in this honorable state.[1] "Say! The truth has come and falsehood has vanished."[2]

As for the science of religion, its glory has **[2a]** become manifest and continues, and the one who cultivates it becomes noble. Its high standing has persisted, its principles have been established, and the seeker is pleased by the time devoted to it. All of this has resulted from the most brilliant supervision [coming] from the most eminent position [the one] held by the Master of Viziers, the Ruler of Men, al-Ṣāḥib, Descendant of [Venerable] Forefathers, Muftī of the Two Parties,[3] Ṣafī l-Dīn 'Abd Allāh ibn 'Alī. May the stars continue to be obedient to his wishes and the crowns of kings continue to bow in his presence as long as the sun rises and rain-bearing, flowing clouds cover the sky. No one can prevent what al-Ṣāḥib desires. He is the sea of sciences whose flow does not abate. He is the full moon of glory whose light is not eclipsed, the lamp of munificence whose flame does not go out, the cloud of generosity whose rain does not cease. He reached **[2b]** the highest perfection and will never be equalled. He rose to the peak of attainment and has no rival. He is unique in his age and the main gemstone in the necklace of glory. If a poetic pun were addressed to him, it would read:

> Whenever a banner was raised in glory, your right and left
> (*yasār*) hands received it.

---

[1] I.e., the Ayyūbid dynasty.

[2] Qur'ān, 17:81; Arberry, *Koran Interpreted*, I, 311.

[3] I.e., the Mālikī and Shāfi'ī law schools that then dominated Egypt.

Whenever a raid was launched on poverty, through you
riches and wealth (also *yasār*) followed.

He gathered [in himself] the merits scattered [among other men but not found all in one man] and ruled free men with determination and firmness. How well the saying goes: "You were created without peer and are above, and the humans and *jinn*[4] are below, the sun of faith rising in the sky of his face and the miracles of its light guide the way to the demise of error." His guidance and visage loom on the horizon of darkness. His finest deeds [stand out above mankind] like Islam stands out above other religions. His dazzling wonders are countless and unlimited, and the memory of them is unforgettable and inconcealable. Human faculties are unable to grasp his excellent qualities, and acknowledge their inability either to carry out the necessary praise of him or to do enough other things to glorify him.

Concerning this I say:

If we spend our lives and traverse ages and eras praising you,
If we exert ourselves with all our might in order to hear and see everything concerning you,
If we adopt the expressions and meanings in poetry and prose and investigate and consider them,
[3a] Then we would learn that speaking of this would be endless and could not be summarized,
Oh, al-Ṣāḥib the King, who has gained such esteem, mastery, and glory?
May your power, high position, and good fortune be everlasting and have no equal.

The respected al-Ṣāḥib, may God exalt him, is the best of those who forgive and the noblest of those who avoid injustice, for he has pardoned and forgiven.

As for the science of the body—his (al-Ṣāḥib's?) goal in this, may God preserve him, by giving him excellent health, allowing him to achieve his promises, improving his condition and transmitting [God's] glory through him in this noble (Ayyūbid) state, the ultimate glory of which is to reveal the science of the body in the manner in which the science of religion was revealed[5]—it is a science by which the conditions of the hu-

[4] Invisible beings, harmful or helpful, that interfere with the lives of mortals; see *EI*^{2}, *s.v.* "Djinn" (D.B. Macdonald/[H. Massé] *et al.*).

[5] The syntactical structure of this aside is awkward and could be translated in several ways.

man body, the actions of which [include] those things required in order to obey God, are known. That is because God, praise be to Him, created for His servants medications of every description that will rid them of illnesses. He also gave man reason as a tool with which to discover those things that benefit him. He taught him to discover medications by means of the art of medicine. He provided animals, which are not endowed with reason, with the [instinctive] knowledge they need of medication. Hence you can see that animals know useful medications without being taught them. [For example,] the stag draws the asp out from its den by sniffing for it until he dislodges it and forces it to expose itself. Then he begins to eat it. While doing so, it bites the stag's lips, **[3b]** but he does not worry. After eating it, he promptly turns to river crayfish, which he eats immediately after devouring the asp, in order to prevent injury from the poison of the snake. The crayfish serve as an antidote. Then, he patiently experiences a terrible thirst. He long endures the excessive thirst, knowing that if he drinks cold water immediately after the asp bite, he would die. He approaches the water, but looks at it from a distance and does not drink for fear of dying. This is an inspiration from God, praise be to Him.[6]

I read in the treatise of al-Tamīmī[7] that if a *saqanqūr*[8] bites a man, it precedes him to water or urinates and wallows in it. If the *saqanqūr* precedes him to water or urinates and wallows in it, the man will die. If the bitten man does so first, then the *saqanqūr* will die. [I also read in it that] if a wolf steps on the onion plant,[9] his feet become numb and he cannot move. The fox therefore takes the onion and uses it to protect himself, fearful that a wolf might come to his pups and eat them. I read

---

[6] The assertion that some animals use other animals or certain plants as antidotes may not be as farfetched as it sounds. See Kim A. McDonald, "Primates and Other Animals Use Wild Plants for Medicinal Purposes Researchers Discover," *The Chronicle of Higher Education*, 19 Feb. 1992, pp. A9 and A12; Richard W. Wrangham and Jane Goodall, "Chimpanzee Use of Medicinal Leaves," in *Understanding Chimpanzees*, ed. Paul G. Heltne and Linda A. Marquardt (Cambridge, Massachusetts: Harvard Univiversity Press, 1989), pp. 22–37.

[7] On Abū 'Abd Allāh Muḥammad ibn Aḥmad ibn Sa'īd al-Tamīmī (d. 380/990), see *GAL* I, 237 and *S* I, 422; *GAS* III, 317–18; Ullmann, *Medizin*, pp. 269–70, index. On al-Tamīmī's *al-Risāla*, which is being referred to here, see Dietrich, *Medicinalia*, p. 196 n. 3; Ullmann, *Medizin*, p. 332.

[8] A kind of lizard, skink: al-Kindī, p. 297; Dietrich, *Medicinalia*, p. 196 n. 4; Steingass, p. 687; Kazimirski, I, 1109. The skink itself was used to make an aphrodisiac and apparently the medieval wonder-drug theriac, which was used as an antidote for poison, among other things; see Leiser and Dols, "Evliyā Chelebi's Description of Medicine," pt. 2, p. 64 n. 10

[9] *Ishqīl*: *Tuhfa*, p. 17; al-Kindī, p. 230.

in the *Ṭabīʿiyyāt al-Shifāʾ* of Ibn Sīnā[10] that if the cheetah consumes the drug known as wolfsbane,[11] he hastens to human dung, eats it, and is cured; and that if a turtle eats a snake, afterwards it eats wild thyme.[12] There are many examples of this kind of thing.

By means of the art of medicine, benefits are attained and harm is avoided. The physician must be very sensitive, highly perceptive, **[4a]** clever, of sharp mind, clear thinking, of good repute, truthful, sincere to whomever asks his advice, well experienced, and well read. Galen mentions in *al-Mayāmir*,[13] in the chapter on medical assistance, that the doctor must possess four qualities. First, he must have piety combined with astuteness, religion (faith) and understanding. Second, he must have knowledge of, and experience with, the natures of the illnesses that he treats. Third, he must have knowledge of, and experience with, the natures of the sick people whom he treats. And fourth, he must have knowledge of, and experience with, the efficacy of medications (i.e., drugs). It is an exalted occupation and experts hold it in high esteem.

I read in a book on the art of medicine by Ibn al-Jawzī[14] where he says, speaking of Shīth ibn Ādam,[15] upon them be peace, that he inherited medicine from Ādam and made it known. He also says: "Abū Saʿīd Aḥmad ibn Muḥammad[16] related to us in a chain of authorities

---

[10] On Ibn Sīnā or Avicenna (d. 428/1037), see *GAL* I, 452–58 and *S* I, 812–28; *EI* [2], *s.v.* "Ibn Sīnā" (A.-M. Goichon); Ullmann, *Medizin*, pp. 152–56; *Dictionary of Scientific Biography*, *s.v.* "Ibn Sīnā" (G.C. Anawati and A.Z. Iskandar). His *Ṭabīʿiyyāt al-Shifāʾ* ["The Natural Sciences (section of the Book of) Healing"] is in course of publication, ed. Ibrāhīm Madkūr, Cairo: al-Maṭbaʿa al-Amīriyya, 1956–proceeding).

[11] *Khāniq al-nimr*: see Edward William Lane, *An Arabic-English Lexicon* (1863–93; repr. Beirut, Librairie du Liban, 1968), I.2, 818.

[12] *Ṣaʿtar*: al-Kindī, p. 297.

[13] On Galen (d. *ca.* AD 199), see *GAL S* III, index; *GAS* III, 68–140; Ullmann, *Medizin*, pp. 35–68, index; Bayard Dodge, trans., *The Fihrist of al-Nadīm* (New York: Columbia University Press, 1970), II, 680–86; *EI* [2], *s.v.* "Djālīnūs" (Richard Walzer); Owsei Temkin, *Galenism: The Rise and Decline of a Medical Philosophy* (Ithaca: Cornell University Press, 1973). On his *al-Mayāmir* ["The Homilies"], the Arabic of which has not been published, see *GAS* III, 119–20, index; Ullmann, *Medizin*, pp. 48, 211.

[14] On Abū l-Farash ʿAbd al-Raḥmān ibn ʿAlī ibn Muḥammed ibn al-Jawzī (d. 597/1200), see *GAL* I, 500–506 and *S* I, 914–20; Dietrich, *Medicinalia*, pp. 110–12; Ullmann, *Medizin*, p. 186; *EI* [2], *s.v.* "Ibn al-Djawzī" (H. Laoust). The book in question is apparently his *Kitāb Luqaṭ al-manāfiʿ fī l-ṭibb* ["The Book of Useful Facts on Medicine"]; Dietrich, *Medicinalia*, p. 197.

[15] I.e., Seth the son of Adam; *EI* [2], *s.v.* "Shīth" (Cl. Huart-[C.E. Bosivorth]).

[16] Apparently Abū Saʿīd Aḥmad ibn Muḥammad ibn Saʿīd al-Nīsābūrī (d. 353/964). See al-Dhahabī, *Tadhkirat al-ḥuffāẓ*, 3rd rev. ed. (Hyderabad, Deccan: Dāʾirat al-Maʿārif al-ʿUthmāniyya, 1375–77/1955–58), III, 920; al-Subkī, *Ṭabaqāt*, III, 43.

going back to Saʿīd ibn Jubayr[17] on the authority of Ibn ʿAbbās[18] on the authority of the Prophet, God bless him and grant him salvation, that Muḥammad said that whenever Soloman son of David, peace be upon him, prayed, he saw a tree standing firmly in front of him. So he would ask it: 'What is your name?' If it were for planting, it would be planted. If it were for a drug, it would be recorded." It is reported too that Usāma ibn Sharīk[19] said: "I was with the Prophet, God bless him and grant him salvation, when some Bedouins came and said: 'Oh, Messenger of God, should we treat ourselves with medicine?' and he replied: 'Yes, Oh, servants of God. Treat yourselves because **[4b]** God, the Powerful and Sublime, did not create any illness without creating for it a cure, except for one thing.' They then asked: 'What was that, Oh, Messenger of God?' And he answered: 'Senility.' "[20]

Al-Aḥnaf ibn Qays[21] said: "There are four things through which a man gains supremacy: knowledge, good manners, integrity, and fidelity. And three that an intelligent man must not put aside: knowledge, which encourages him to work; medicine, which is used to protect his body; and a craft, by which he can earn his living."

It is also reported on the authority of al-Shāfiʿī,[22] may God's mercy be upon him, that he said: "Knowledge is of two kinds: knowledge for religion and knowledge for this world. For the former there is law (*fiqh*) and for the latter there is medicine."[23] It was also reported that al-Shāfiʿī, may God's mercy be upon him, said: "There are two classes of men whom people cannot do without: physicians for their bodies and jurists for their religion." It was said that an intelligent man should not live in a town that does not have five things: a just ruler, a

---

[17] On Saʿīd ibn Jubayr al-Wālibī (d. *ca.* 95/714), see al-Dhahabī, *Tadhkirat*, I, 76–77.

[18] On ʿAbd Allāh ibn al-ʿAbbās (d. 68/687–88), see *EI*², *s.v.* " ʿAbd Allāh ibn al-ʿAbbās" (L. Veccia Vaglieri).

[19] On Usāma ibn Sharīk al-Ṣaḥābī (d. *ca.* 70/689–90), see al-Ṣafadī, *al-Wāfī*, VIII, 375. For this *ḥadīth*, see A.J. Wensinck, *A Handbook of Early Muhammadan Tradition* (Leiden: E.J. Brill, 1960), p. 148.

[20] On these *ḥadīths*, see J.C. Bürgel, "Secular and Religious Features of Medieval Arabic Medicine," in *Asian Medical Systems: A Comparative Study*, ed. Charles Leslie (Berkeley: University of California Press, 1976), pp. 55–56. The *ḥadīth* in which the Prophet states that there was no cure for senility expresses an ancient sentiment. It is found, for example, at the beginning of Aristophanes' (448?–380? BC) *Lysistrata* (Norwalk, Connecticut: The Easton Press, 1983), p. 25.

[21] On al-Aḥnaf (d. 72/691–92), see *EI*², *s.v.* "al-Aḥnaf b. Ḳays" (Ch. Pellat).

[22] On Abū ʿAbd Allāh Muḥammad ibn Idrīs al-Shāfiʿī (d. 204/820), see *EI*², *s.v.* "al-Shāfiʿī" (E. Chaumont).

[23] On this often repeated *ḥadīth*, see Bürgel, "Medieval Arabic Medicine," p. 56.

learned judge, an expert physician, an established market, and a flowing river.

As for the practitioners of this art under the administration (*maqām*) of al-Ṣāḥib, may God exalt it, he has eliminated harmful elements by preventing whomever claims to know it but does not have the qualifications or superior knowledge [from practicing it], for this art is multifaceted, unrestricted, has countless procedures, and is fraught with dangers and perils. The barber cupper treats illnesses of the eye and wounds, and the ophthalmologist treats illnesses of the body, because these fields are open to anyone who wishes to enter them.

So may God have mercy on 'Abd al-'Azīz (the author). He has won much praise and a fine reputation during his short term in office. And he wished al-Ṣāḥib, who had appointed him, a long life. **[5a]** It was the practice of this slave to serve the honorable and excellent al-Ṣāḥib, may God exalt him, in a profession that is studied and not forgotten because it is transferred from written lines to the breasts of men. He too followed this path and wrote this concise work so that one can ascertain with it the knowledge of someone who claims to know this art and how much he understands, and reveal the quality of his knowledge and practice. I divided my treatise into ten chapters, each containing twenty questions that not a single physician will be able to answer unless he studies them and remembers them. I only mentioned what is well known and set down in writing. Then, I mentioned the answer for each question and the place from which I took it, so that this will be an authoritative source for the questioner in case the respondent gives him a different answer. It can, therefore, be said to the respondent that a given question has been recorded, that so and so mentioned it in such and such a book in such and such a place. My only intention here is to make a collection of these questions gathered from the books of our predecessors. I entitled it *The Experts' Examination for All Physicians*. May God, praise be to Him the Exalted, forever grant me success in the service of al-Ṣāḥib's administration and place me among those of whom God said: "They will rejoice in mercy from Him and good pleasure."[24]

CHAPTER ONE is on the Pulse and Understanding It
CHAPTER TWO is on the Urine and What It Reveals
CHAPTER THREE is on Fevers and Crises
CHAPTER FOUR is on Favorable and Dangerous Symptoms
[5b] CHAPTER FIVE is on Simple Drugs
CHAPTER SIX is on Treatment

---

24 Cf. Qur'ān, 9:21; Arberry, *Koran Interpreted*, I, 209.

CHAPTER SEVEN is on What the Ophthalmologist Should be Asked
CHAPTER EIGHT is on What Surgeons Should Know
CHAPTER NINE is on What the Bonesetter Should be Asked
CHAPTER TEN is on the Fundamentals of This Art

CHAPTER ONE

ON THE PULSE, COMPRISING TWENTY QUESTIONS

QUESTION ONE: Is it possible for a doctor to deduce the name of a lover from the pulse? How is this possible?

ANSWER: This is recorded in the *Juz'iyyāt* of Ibn Sīnā's *al-Qānūn*, where he says: Love is a psychological illness. With regard to this, the pulse fluctuates irregularly like the pulse of someone suffering from anxiety, so that one can tell from it the name of the beloved. The way to do this is to mention many names while the hand is on the pulse. If it fluctuates greatly at the mention of a certain person, describe his appearance and features and repeat his name. If the fluctuation in pulse rate increases and begins to seem disrupted, then you know the name of the beloved.[1]

QUESTION TWO: How many things **[6a]** does someone trained in the pulse need to determine?

ANSWER: Five. This is recorded in the fifth treatise of Galen's *al-Nabḍ al-kabīr*,[2] where he says: The first thing a physician needs to discover concerning the pulse is the extent of its expansion (diastole); second, the duration of movement; third, the condition of the [vital] faculty[3] that activates the pulsating vein (artery); fourth, the condition of the dermis of the vein and its throbbing; fifth, he needs to know the duration of the pause.

QUESTION THREE: How many pairings occur in the pulse when the cause of change is [bodily] need and the [vital] faculty? What happens to the pulse?

---

[1] Ibn Sīnā's monumental medical work, *al-Qānūn fī l-ṭibb* ["The Canon of Medicine"], is roughly divided into two parts, generalities (*kulliyyāt*) and specifics (*juz'iyyāt*). For this passage, see *al-Qānūn*, II, 72; Michael Dols, *Majnūn: The Madman in Medieval Islamic Society* (Oxford: Oxford University Press, 1992), pp. 90–91, 484.

[2] Al-Sulamī also refers to it as *Kitāb al-Nabḍ al-kabīr* ["The Great Book on the Pulse"], the Arabic of which has not been published. See *GAS* III, 91–94; Ullmann, *Medizin*, pp. 43, 90. On this answer, cf. Ḥunayn, p. 71.

[3] The entire physiological process was governed by the interaction of various faculties. The "vital" or "animal" faculties ensured life and were manifest in the systole and diastole of the heart and arteries. See Manfred Ullmann, *Islamic Medicine* (Edinburgh: Edinburgh University Press, 1978), pp. 60–62.

ANSWER: Four. This is recorded in the ninth treatise of Galen's *Kitāb al-Nabḍ al-kabīr*, where he says: First, when the [vital] faculty is very weak [combined] with a rise in [innate] heat[4] making the pulse very slight, slow, and strained; second, a weak [vital] faculty [combined] with a lukewarm innate heat and its weakness makes the pulse sluggish because of the dwindling [vital] faculty. The slightness and slowness resemble the first pairing but without the extreme degree of regularity. Third, when the [vital] faculty and [innate] heat increase together making the pulse extremely strong and large but not very fast; and fourth, when a correct [vital] faculty and a lack of [innate] heat make the pulse of moderate magnitude and very **[6b]** slow with great irregularity, especially if coldness increases significantly.

QUESTION FOUR: How is it known that the pulse has a musical nature?

ANSWER: This is recorded in Ibn Sīnā's *al-Kulliyyāt*, where he says: Just as the art of music is brought about by the composition of melodies according to sharpness and dullness [of sounds] and in certain rhythmic intervals between which lie the beats, so the same situation holds for the pulse. Thus, measure of time in this situation regarding speed and regularity is rhythmical and the measure of its conditions regarding strength and weakness is like a composition. And just as the periods of rhythm and range of melodies can be harmonious or disharmonious and likewise the disparities can be regular or irregular, so the measures of the conditions of the pulse concerning strength, weakness, and range (i.e., amount) can be harmonious or disharmonious.[5]

QUESTION FIVE: How many things are taken into consideration when determining the similarity of the components of a pulse beat, or one component of a pulse beat?

ANSWER: This is recorded in Ibn Sīnā's *al-Kulliyyāt*. There are five things: largeness and smallness, strength and weakness, speed and slowness, irregularity and regularity, and hardness and softness.[6]

---

[4] "Innate heat" was the central element of life and was contained in the heart. See Ullmann, *Islamic Medicine*, pp. 65, 67.

[5] *Al-Qānūn*, I, 125. Cf. O. Cameron Gruner, *A Treatise on the Canon of Medicine of Avicenna* (1930; repr. New York: August M. Kelly, 1970), p. 292. This translation of the first book of *al-Qānūn* is useful, but, as a strict translation, it should be used with caution. It is based on the Latin version of this work. A better translation of the first book based on the Arabic text is Mazhar H. Shah's *General Principles of Avicenna's Canon of Medicine* (Karachi, Pakistan: Naveed Clinic, 1966), cf. p. 236.

[6] *Al-Qānūn*, I, 125. Cf. Gruner, *Canon*, pp. 290–91; Shah, *Principles*, p. 236.

QUESTION SIX: **[7a]** How does sleeping on a full or empty stomach affect the pulse, and how is it affected when one is awakened naturally or by something externally?

ANSWER: This is recorded in Ibn Sīnā's *al-Kulliyyāt*, where he says: The pulse changes its features according to the time of sleep and the state of digestion. At the beginning of sleep, the pulse is small and weak because the movement of the innate heat at that time makes it contract and withdraw rather than expand and rise [to the surface]. This is because at that time the [innate] heat is directed by the actions of the life [force] completely to the interior in order to digest the food and ripen the remnant (waste). Then the pulse becomes slower and irregular because the innate heat, even if an increase occurs in it because of retention [of food], lacks the increase [in temperature] that it had during the state of awakening caused by the warming movement [resulting from activity]. If the food becomes digestible during sleep, the pulse returns and becomes strong as a result of the increase in the [vital] faculty from the food and the passing [back to the surface] of what [heat] had gone to the interior to regulate nourishment. So the pulse becomes strong. If sleep continues for some time, the pulse returns but is weak, because of the retention of the innate heat and the suppression of the [vital] faculty under the remnants, which must be emptied by various means while awake, such as by exercise and [various forms of] evacuation. If sleep coincides from the beginning with an empty stomach, smallness, slowness, and irregularity will continue in the pulse. If one wakes up naturally, the pulse gradually tends to become strong and fast. If **[7b]** one wakes up suddenly, this makes the pulse large and irregular to [the extent of] trembling. Then it quickly returns to normal.[7]

QUESTION SEVEN: What causes a diffused pulse?

ANSWER: This is recorded in Ibn Sīnā's *al-Kulliyyāt*, where he says: The cause of a diffused pulse is the variation in the crudity, unripeness, and ripeness of what pours through the body (i.e., inside the walls) of the veins; the difference in the conditions of the veins in hardness and softness; and the inflamation in the nervous (or sinewy) organs.[8] Regarding this, Ibn al-Tilmīdh[9] says: The cause of the diffusion of the pulse for someone with pleurisy and the like is not what Ibn Sīnā mentioned.

---

[7] *Al-Qānūn*, I, 132–33. Cf. Gruner, *Canon*, pp. 315–17; Shah, *Principles*, pp. 249–50.

[8] *Al-Qānūn*, I, 129. Cf. Gruner, *Canon*, p. 306; Shah, *Principles*, p. 243.

[9] On Abū l-Ḥasan Hibat Allāh ibn Sa'īd ibn al-Tilmīdh (d. 560/1165), see *GAL* I, 488 and *S* I, 891; Dietrich, *Medicinalia*, pp. 106–107, 231–32; Ullmann, *Medizin*, pp. 163, *et passim*; *EI* [2], *s.v.* "Ibn al-Tilmīdh" (Max Meyerhof).

Instead, it is the rise in [certain] components [of the pulse] because of [bodily] need, the decline in [certain] components [of the pulse] because of pain, and the irritation this causes in the arteries that pulsate in the same inflamation. Then, these different movements spread to the rest of the arteries, because the cause of the diastole and that which is agitated by harm is the same, that is, the vital faculty.

QUESTION EIGHT: Why does the pulse of someone with watery dropsy tend to be hard?

ANSWER: This is recorded in Galen's *al-Nabḍ al-kabīr*, where he says: The pulse of someone with watery dropsy tends to be hard because a large amount of moisture collects in it from what is contained in the stomach. This moisture may harm the arteries by association. Thus, it causes a distention of the vein and makes it incline toward hardness. **[8a]** Moreover, because of the harm and injury to the [vital] faculty and the coldness of the vein, the pulse becomes small. The smaller the pulse, the more regular it is, especially if it is accompanied by a fever.

QUESTION NINE: How is the pulse of someone with jaundice who has no fever and why is it like that?

ANSWER: This is recorded in the thirteenth treatise of Galen's *al-Nabḍ al-kabīr*, where he says: The pulse of someone with jaundice who has no fever is small, hard, and very regular but neither weak nor fast. As for why it is like that, he says: Because it is in the nature of the yellow bile to dry like dry salt water. For this reason, it makes the dermis of the vein drier and harder. As for the smallness, it occurs because the rigid organ (i.e., the substance of the vessel) is not able to fully expand. Thus, the degree of its regularity corresponds to the degree of its smallness. It is not weak because the [vital] faculty is not weak, and it is not fast because there is no fever. If there were a fever, the pulse would be fast because of [bodily] need.[10]

QUESTION TEN: What are well-balanced, normal, divergent, and deviate pulses?

ANSWER: This is recorded in the first treatise of Galen's *al-Nabḍ al-kabīr*, where he says: The vein of a person of any age is in a certain natural balance. If this balance remains with him, **[8b]** it is called well balanced. If it departs from him slightly and the departure of the natural balance corresponds to the balance of someone whose age is close to that of the patient, it is called normal. If it does not correspond to that of someone

[10] Cf. Ḥunayn, p. 7.

whose age is close to that of the patient but to any another age, it is called divergent. If the pulse does not correspond to that of any age, it is called deviate.

QUESTION ELEVEN: What do you say about pulses that are well balanced and poorly balanced, standard and divergent, and regular and irregular, with respect to the types according to which they are classified?

ANSWER: There are four types. This is recorded in the seventh treatise of *al-Malakī*, where the author says: The well-balanced and poorly balanced, standard and divergent, and regular and irregular pulses only exist in four types. They are the types based on the amount of the diastole, the manner of movement, the amount of the [vital] faculty, and the duration of the pause. There are no possibilities other than these four types.[11]

QUESTION TWELVE: Between the standard and divergent pulse, is there an average as there is between large and small or fast and slow?

ANSWER: There is no average between them. This is recorded in the seventh treatise of *al-Juz' al-ʿamalī* of *al-Malakī*, where the author says: There **[9a]** is no median between the standard and divergent pulse because the standard pulse is normal and healthy while the divergent is abnormal and does not occur unless one is ill, so the median between them is not standard.[12]

QUESTION THIRTEEN: In which body is the pulse greater, a naturally frail body or a plump body, and why?

ANSWER: This is recorded in *al-Malakī*, where the author says: The pulse is greater and stronger in frail bodies than in plump, very fleshy bodies. The pulse of a plump body is smaller and weaker because the artery in a plump body conceals it and weighs heavily on it because of the large amound of flesh. The pulse of a plump body, however, is more regular as a result of the decline in the [vital] faculty [coming] from the enlarged artery, making the regularity compensate for the largeness.[13]

---

11 This is from ʿAlī ibn al-ʿAbbās al-Majūsī's (d. between 372/982 and 386/995) *Kāmil al-ṣināʿa al-ṭibbiyya* ["The Complete Medical Art"] or *al-Malakī* ["The Royal Book"]. For this answer, see *al-Malakī*, I, 262. On the author, known as Haly Abbas in the West, and this work, see *GAL* I, 238 and *S* I, 423; *GAS* III, 320–22; Dietrich, *Medicinalia*, pp. 61–63; Ullmann, *Medizin*, pp. 140–46, index; *EI* 2, *s.v.* " ʿAlī b. al-ʿAbbās" (C. Elgood).

12 *Al-Malakī*, I, 263.

13 *Ibid.*, I, 264.

QUESTION FOURTEEN: How is the pulse of a pregnant woman, and why is it like that?

ANSWER: This is recorded in *al-Malakī*. The pulse of a pregnant woman is large and extremely fast and regular because the [innate] heat of her body is high as a result of what is added to her temperament from the heat of the fetus. Its heat is carried to the arteries of the woman by the connection of the arteries of the fetus in the placenta to her arteries. However, in the sixth month, her pulse becomes weak and slow.[14]

QUESTION FIFTEEN: What is the special pulse of each kind of **[9b]** dropsy?

ANSWER: This is recorded in Ibn Sīnā's *al-Qānūn*, where he says: As for ascites, the pulse is small, regular, and tends to be hard and a bit distended because of the distention of the membranes. Sometimes toward the end, it tends to be soft because of the excess of moisture. As for anasarca, the pulse is throbbing, wide, and soft. As for *ṭablī* (drum-like, bulging, in which the navel protrudes), the pulse is long but not weak.[15]

QUESTION SIXTEEN: How is the pulse of someone who suffers from anxiety?

ANSWER: This is recorded in *al-Malakī*. Small, weak, and irregular. If it (the anxiety) continues until it consumes the [vital] faculty, the pulse becomes worm-like and then ant-like (i.e., increasingly faint) while the [vital] faculty declines and disappears.[16]

QUESTION SEVENTEEN: How is the pulse of someone suffering from diphtheria, and what are the symptoms of the transformation of the substance of it (this illness) into pneumonia or moving in the direction of the heart from the pulse?

ANSWER: This is recorded in Ibn Sīnā's *al-Qānūn*. As for the pulse of someone who has just come down with diphtheria, it is regular and divergent. Then it becomes small and irregular. If the pulse throbs greatly and coughing starts, then the illness is turning to pneumonia. If the pulse becomes extremely weak, small and irregular; and if the heart begins to palpitate and the innate nature [of the body] dissolves; and if fainting occurs, then the substance is flowing in the direction of the heart.[17]

---

14 *Ibid.*, I, 266.

15 *Al-Qānūn*, II, 388–89.

16 *Al-Malakī*, I, 269.

17 *Al-Qānūn*, II, 200–201.

QUESTION EIGHTEEN: How does pleasure affect the pulse?

ANSWER: **[10a]** This is recorded in the twelfth treatise of Galen's *al-Nabḍ al-kabīr*, where he says: Pleasure makes the pulse large, irregular and slow.

QUESTION NINETEEN: Which causes dread, an extremely hard pulse or an extremely soft pulse?

ANSWER: Both of them equally. This is recorded in the fourteenth treatise of Galen's *al-Nabḍ al-kabīr*, where he says: As for an extremely hard pulse, it makes one fear the consequences with no sense of assurance, like an extremely soft pulse, because the extreme hardness results from plethora, or a large inflamation in some of the intestines, or from the immobility resulting from coldness, or from the dryness resulting from an ardent fever or very strong convulsions. The extremely soft pulse results from very excessive moisture.

QUESTION TWENTY: How is the pulse if an inflamation festers?

ANSWER: This is recorded in the twelfth treatise of Galen's *al-Nabḍ al-kabīr*, where he says: The pulse is divergent and irregular because of the harm the organ suffers and the decline in the [vital] faculty and the resistance of nature to, and its struggle against, the illness.

CHAPTER TWO

ON URINE, COMPRISING TWENTY QUESTIONS

[10b] QUESTION ONE: If thin colorless urine appears on the fourth day of an illness and bad symptoms follow it, what would be your prognosis?

ANSWER: This is recorded in *al-Malakī*, where the author says: When this urine appears with bad symptoms on the fourth day, the patient will die before the seventh.[1]

QUESTION TWO: What does thin yellow urine indicate?

ANSWER: This is recorded in *al-Malakī*, where the author says: It indicates that the weakness of the nature does not allow the substance [of the illness] to ripen properly. The nature started to ripen the substance and began with the color, changing it to yellow, for nature begins with ripening[2] the color because it is easier. Then it starts to ripen the body [of the substance].[3]

QUESTION THREE: If viscous[4] colorless urine appears on a day of crisis, especially the fourth day, what does this indicate?

ANSWER: This is recorded in al-Isrā'īlī's *Kitāb al-Bawl*,[5] where he says: It indicates the end of pains of the joints and inflamations appearing at the base of the ears. If it appears after the crisis, it indicates a return of the illness. God knows best.

QUESTION FOUR: If viscous urine persists and does not change for a long time, what does this indicate?

---

[1] *Al-Malakī*, I, 284. It is worthy of note that the distinction between a medical prognosis based on an analysis of urine and outright urinomancy could be vague. The Arabs themselves poked fun at this. For a parody of urine analysis, see, for example, "The Tale of the Weaver who Became a Leach by Order of his Wife," in Richard Burton, trans., *Supplemental Nights to the Book of the Thousand Nights and a Night* (Benares = Stoke Newington, London, 1886–88), I, 194–98.

[2] On ripening, see below, Chapter 10, Question 8.

[3] *Al-Malakī*, I, 284. Cf. Ḥunayn, p. 97.

[4] Viscosity in a substance generally implies that there is something crude or morbid in it.

[5] On Abū Ya'qūb Isḥāq ibn Sulaymān al-Isrā'īlī (d. *ca.* 320/932) and his *Kitāb al-Bawl* ["Book on Urine"], which has not been published, see *GAL* I, 236 and *S* I, 421; *GAS* III, 295–97; Dietrich, *Medicinalia*, pp. 239–40; Ullmann, *Medizin*, pp. 137–38; *EI*², *s.v.* "Isḥāḳ b. Sulaymān al-Isrā'īlī" (A. Altman).

ANSWER: **[11a]** This is recorded in al-Isrā'īlī's *Kitāb al-Bawl*, where he says: This indicates an inflamation has occurred in the hypochondrium. If favorable symptoms follow it, this indicates recovery, otherwise dangerous consequences are to be feared.

QUESTION FIVE: What does fine red urine with a pungent odor and black sediment that causes a hairlike cloudiness indicate?

ANSWER: This is recorded in al-Isrā'īlī's book on the urine, where he says: This is bad and dangerous consequences are to be feared.

QUESTION SIX: What does unclear viscous urine accompanied by deafness, a headache, and a distention of the anterior wall of the abdomen indicate?

ANSWER: This is recorded in al-Isrā'īlī's book, where he says: This indicates that a bad case of jaundice will occur before the seventh day. If the urine becomes fine and there is something dull-colored suspended in it, and the rest of the symptoms are similar [to those mentioned], this indicates a relapse and a dullness of the mind, especially if the patient is a heavy eater.

QUESTION SEVEN: What does a small amount of pure red urine accompanied by dropsy indicate?

ANSWER: This is recorded in al-Isrā'īlī's book, where he says: This indicates that death is near.

QUESTION EIGHT: What do blood-red urine accompanied by vomiting something like verdigris, **[11b]** and a rough tongue indicate?

ANSWER: This is recorded in al-Isrā'īlī's book, where he says: This indicates danger and imminent death.

QUESTION NINE: What does blond urine with a foam like that of wine indicate?

ANSWER: It indicates mental complications.[6]

QUESTION TEN: What does black urine indicate when it is thin from the beginning of an illness?

ANSWER: This is recorded in *al-Malakī*, where the author says: It indicates certain death.[7]

---

6 Dols, *Majnūn*, p. 69.

7 *Al-Malakī*, I, 285. Cf. Hippocrates, *Hippocratic Writings*, trans. Francis Adams in *Great Books of the Western World*, ed. Robert Maynard Hutchins (Chicago: Encyclopaedia Britannica, 1952), X, 22; *Hippocratic Writings*, trans. J. Chadwick *et al.* (Harmondsworth, UK: Penguin Books, 1983), p. 176.

QUESTION ELEVEN: How many kinds of residual sediments are there?

ANSWER: This is recorded in *al-Malakī*, where the author says: There are three. The first is cloudy. It is what appears at the top of the urine flask. The second is suspended. It is what appears in the middle [of the flask]. And the third is the deposit that appears at the bottom [of the flask].[8]

QUESTION TWELVE: What does a persistent green urine with a flaming or gentle fever indicate?

ANSWER: It is recorded by al-Isrā'īlī that if it accompanies a flaming fever, it indicates complications. If it accompanies a gentle fever, for which the patient has drunk insufficient water, it indicates a wasting away (i.e., dehydration) of the body.

QUESTION THIRTEEN: **[12a]** What does fine black urine, in which there are black particles that do not sink but float, accompanied by a flaming fever, insomnia, and deafness indicate?

ANSWER: This is recorded by al-Isrā'īlī. It indicates a protracted illness that terminates by an emission of blood.

QUESTION FOURTEEN: What does black urine, in which there is granular separated sediment similar to drops, accompanied by an inflamation and pain in the anterior wall of the abdomen, indicate?

ANSWER: This is recorded by al-Isrā'īlī, where he says: This indicates death.

QUESTION FIFTEEN: If black thin urine changes to blond and viscous and no odor accompanies it, what does this indicate?

ANSWER: This is recorded in Ibn Sīnā's *al-Juz'iyyāt*, where he says: This indicates an illness in the liver, especially jaundice, because this change to viscous from thin and to blond from black indicates either a loss of [innate] heat and the occurrence of digestion, and what accompanies or follows this is lightness in color. If this is not the case, it indicates that a substance has lodged in the liver without being purified, thus causing the blackness. If it becomes hot, it would seem to you that it has caused an inflamation.[9]

QUESTION SIXTEEN: **[12b]** What does viscous urine that is not clear indicate?

---

[8] *Al-Malakī*, I, 285–86. Cf. Hippocrates, *Hippocratic Writings*, Adams trans. p. 22, Chadwick *et al.* trans., p. 176; Ḥunayn, p. 96.

[9] *Al-Qānūn*, III, 100.

ANSWER: This is recorded by al-Isrā'īlī, where he says: This indicates that a flatulent coarse gas has mixed with the sediment and stimulated it. Thus, it indicates that a headache is present or will occur.

QUESTION SEVENTEEN: What does very red urine that becomes viscous during exhausting fevers and is followed by the appearance of a lot of sediment that does not settle, which is accompanied by a headache, indicate?

ANSWER: This is recorded in *al-Juz'iyyāt* of Ibn Sīnā's *al-Qānūn*, where he says: This indicates a protracted illness because the substance [of the illness] is resistant and therefore it does not become viscous at first. When it does, it (sediment) does not settle quickly. Its crisis (i.e., that of the illness) occurs in a vein because the substance [of the illness] inclines to the veins. Urine like this resembles [that present in] jaundice but differs from it in that it does not stain clothing.[10]

QUESTION EIGHTEEN: What does dark red urine that passes easily indicate?

ANSWER: This is recorded by al-Isrā'īlī, where he says: This indicates the fever will end after the seventh day.

QUESTION NINETEEN: If the urine has a sour odor and the illness is hot, what does this indicate?

ANSWER: This is recorded in *al-Kulliyyāt*, where the author says: This indicates **[13a]** death because it indicates the extinguishing of the innate heat and a coldness seizing the nature [of the body] together with extraneous heat.[11]

QUESTION TWENTY: How many kinds of abnormal sediments are there?

ANSWER: This is recorded in *al-Kulliyyāt*. There are eighteen (*sic*): flaky, bran-like, vetch-like, like crushed wheat, similar to red arsenic, saturated with yellow, fleshy, mucus-like, greasy, *madī* (a sediment that easily comes together and disperses accompanied by a chronic putridity indicating an inflamation), similar to pieces of yeast, like blood, like clotted blood, hair-like, sandy, like pebbles, and ash-like.[12] God knows best what is correct.

---

10 *Ibid*. Cf. Ḥunayn, p. 104.

11 *Al-Qānūn*, I, 142. Cf. Gruner, *Canon*, p. 338; Shah, *Principles*, p. 266.

12 *Al-Qānūn*, I, 143. Ibn Sīnā does not state a specific number of unnatural sediments. Al-Sulamī's count is somewhat confused. Cf. Gruner, *Canon*, pp. 341–43; Shah, *Principles*, pp. 268–71. Cf. also Ḥunayn, p. 99.

CHAPTER THREE

ON FEVERS AND CRISES, COMPRISING TWENTY QUESTIONS

QUESTION ONE: How many kinds of ephemeral fevers does Ibn Sīnā classify?

ANSWER: Twenty-three. This is recorded in the fourth book of *al-Qānūn*. They are fever from [too much] grief, anxiety, thinking [about something], anger, staying awake, sleeping, resting, joy, fear, tiredness, excreting, pain, fainting, hunger, thirst, an obstruction [of the pores], dyspepsia, [internal] inflamation, being unclean, [innate] heat, **[13b]** contraction [of the pores] from coldness, contraction [of the pores] from alum water, wine drinking, and [hot] food.[1]

QUESTION TWO: How many symptoms are there for tertian fever?

ANSWER: Their number is nineteen. This is recorded in the second treatise of Galen's *Kitāb al-Buḥrān*, where he says: First, strong shivering; second, the flesh feels as if it were being pricked by needles; third, at the beginning of its paroxysms the pulse is small, slow, and irregular, but much less slow and much less irregular than during quartan fever. When it does increase, the speed becomes standard. Fourth, thirst and a burning sensation persist until it ends; fifth, the temperature spreads equally throughout the body; sixth, if you put your hand on the body, you will encounter a great heat as if it were rising with steam. But before long it subsides and your hand will overcome it; seventh, when cold water is drunk, hot steam rises from the patient's body. When it reaches the skin, it oozes as perspiration; eighth, he vomits yellow bile; ninth, but sometimes different kinds of bile are produced and his urine becomes **[14a]** mostly bile; tenth, at the beginning the patient's perspiration is steamy and fiery like that given off in the bath; eleventh, the pulse is like that of a healthy person who has just exercised: fast, large, strong, and regular; twelfth, the attack of fever will not last more than twelve hours, which is the longest period possible; thirteenth, the urine becomes radiant yellow, pure red, and has a medium thickness. There can occur on the top of the urine, or suspended in the middle, a floating white cloud; fourteenth, it will not continue for more than seven attacks; fifteenth, the period will

---

[1] *Al-Qānūn*, III, 8–15.

be hot and dry; sixteenth, there will be a burning feeling; seventeenth, the bile will dominate the nature [of the body]; eighteenth, the patient will start to have insomnia, to worry, to be fatigued, and to lose his appetite; and nineteenth, at the present time many people are seized by tertian fever.[2]

QUESTION THREE: How many symptoms are there for quartan fever?

ANSWER: Nine. This is recorded in the second treatise of Galen's *Kitāb al-Buḥrān*, where he says: First, **[14b]** strong shivering is not present at the beginning. Instead, one mostly feels cold. The coldness resembles that to which people are exposed by extremely cold air in the winter. There is something that makes one cold and strikes him until it reaches the bones; second, at the beginning of its paroxysms, the pulse is small, weak, slow, and irregular. It will seem to you in the paroxysms of quartan fever that the perspiration is shackled and blocked, as if it were drawn to the interior and prevented from rising; third, it is more prevelent in the autumn. If the autumn has mixed weather, you can be certain that the fever is quartan; fourth, one should look to see if the [geographic] location is the cause of it; fifth, one should look to see if the nature of the patient tends to be melancholy; sixth, one should look to see if what preceded this has caused the melancholia; seventh, one should look to see if many people were afflicted by it; eighth, one should look to see if the urine is colorless, thin, and watery; and ninth, one should look to see if the patient has a thick spleen or if he once had a complicated fever. Galen said in the same place: Whoever is not able to distinguish between quartan fever and tertian fever from the very first day knows nothing about medicine.[3]

QUESTION FOUR: **[15a]** How many symptoms are there for the fever that occurs every day?

ANSWER: Twelve. This is recorded in the second treatise of Galen's *Kitāb al-Buḥrān*, where he says: First, there is shivering from the first day; second, if it continues for a number of days, the patient exhibits an apparent coldness at the start of the attack; third, a disparity exists in the pulse. It undermines its proper operation at the start of the attack, but it is not like that found in tertian fever with regard to speed, size, and

---

[2] The Arabic text of the *Kitāb al-Buḥrān* ["Book on Crises"] has not been published; see *GAS* III, 95; and Ullmann, *Medizin*, p. 43. For this citation, cf. al-Rāzī, *Kitāb al-Ḥāwī fī l-ṭibb* (Hyderabad, Deccan: Dā'irat al-Ma'ārif al-'Uthmāniyya, 1374–90/1955–70), XV, 94–101.

[3] Cf. al-Rāzī, *al-Ḥāwī*, XVI, 96–99.

strength; fourth, the patient does not have an intense burning sensation nor is his breathing heavy; fifth, the thirst is less than that in other fevers; sixth, the urine on the first day is like that on the first day of quartan fever, but the patient hardly perspires from the first days; seventh, the nature of the body is humid and, thus, it most frequently afflicts children; eighth, there is pain in the stomach and liver; ninth, it will be preceded by indigestion; tenth, the patient has an inflamation in the hypochondrium; eleventh, the patient's complexion is between yellow and white; and twelfth, among those things that affect its occurrence are place of birth and location.[4]

QUESTION FIVE: **[15b]** How many special symptoms are there for ephemeral fever?

ANSWER: Eight. This is recorded in Galen's *Kitāb al-Ḥummayāt*.[5] First is the appearance of ripening in the urine on the first day. Second, if the pulse can increase in size and speed, it does so as much as it can and it is accompanied by regularity. Third, the perspiration declines and there is absolutely no increase in speed. But if it does increase under certain conditions, the increase is very little and its deviation from normal is slight. Fourth, the heat (temperature) is good and pleasant. Fifth, the pulse is standard. Sixth, the fever increases without pressure on the heat or pulse. Seventh, there is a decline of the fever if there is perspiration or moisture or damp steam coming from the body. There follows a complete departure of the fever. And eighth, the cause of it is clear and apparent.

QUESTION SIX: How many special symptoms are there for putrid fever?

ANSWER: Seven. This is recorded in Galen's *Kitāb al-Ḥummayāt*. First, this fever should not be preceded by an obvious cause that can be recognized from the outset. Second, at the beginning, there is shivering without the body being **[16a]** struck beforehand by an excessive sun-like heat or excessive cold. Third, there is a disparity in the pulse. Fourth, there is a disparity in the heat (temperature). Fifth, the quality of the heat is neither pleasurable nor tranquil to the extent of an ephemeral fever. But with regard to a smokey fever, it is similar, so that it is

[4] Cf. *ibid.*, XVI, 52–53.

[5] The Arabic text of this work ["Book on Fevers"] has not been published. Cf. *GAS* III, 94–95; Ullmann, *Medizin*, p. 42; Dodge, *Fihrist*, II, 683. Note also a book with the same title by Ḥunayn ibn Isḥāq, who translated much of Galen into Arabic, *GAS* III, 254.

irritating and stinging to the touch except at the beginning of the attack of the fever. Earlier, the heat was obscure and the stages through which it passed were hidden. Thus, one did not detect it when first touching the body. If the palm of the hand remains on the body for a while, the heat will rise from deep below. Sixth, no trace of ripening is seen in the urine. Seventh, at the time of the attack of the fever, some of the symptoms of an ardent fever appear, or some of the symptoms of the fever that makes the patient feel cold and hot at the same time appear, or some of the symptoms of the fever that is extremely hot inside the body but cold outside appear, or some of the symptoms of semi-tertian fever appear, or some of the symptoms of *lathiqa*[6] fever appear.

QUESTION SEVEN: Why do a fever that is from the decay of yellow bile take one day to come and one day to leave, phlegmatic fever attack every day, and quartan fever take twice as long to leave as it did to come on?

ANSWER: As for what is caused by decay of the yellow bile, heat and dryness combine in it. The nature of heat is one of continuous movement **[16b]** and expansion of the elements. It is the stronger of the two actors while dryness is the stronger of the two things acted upon. It is in the nature of dryness to combine the elements, shrink them, and prevent what causes the heat. To prevent dryness from resulting from the continuation of the action of the heat, this fever comes one day and leaves the next. As for the attacking fever, each day the coldness and humidity meet. It is in the nature of coldness to combine and contract. It is in the nature of humidity to expand and separate. During decay, humidity will predominate. Thus the attack of this fever is not prolonged. On any day, its departure will take six hours, which is a quarter of a day. Sometimes it is less than that or more. As for quartan fever, it is caused by black bile. Coldness and dryness combine in it. Coldness is the weaker of the two actors and less active. Dryness is the stronger of the two things acted upon. Because of the participation of coldness and dryness in combining and contracting and in repose and minimal movement, the attack of the illness is not delayed while the period of the attack is delayed until the [time of the] departure of the attack takes twice as long as it did to come on.

QUESTION EIGHT: How many courses may a patient's illness take during a crisis?[7]

---

6 Dozy, II, 524, pituitous and continuous.

7 A "crisis" was a condition in which a disease suddenly took a turn for the worse

ANSWER: Six. This is recorded in the third treatise of Galen's *al-Buḥrān*, where he says: The patient's illness may take six courses. His momentum may move towards good health and this is called an absolute crisis; or he dies and this is called a fatal crisis; or his progress may move **[17a]** little by little towards good health, that is, the illness diminishes bit by bit, and the patient is said to recover; or he may give in little by little, that is, the strength of the patient ebbs, which is called a crisis of decline; or both processes may occur together, leading to good health; or both processes may occur together, leading to death.

QUESTION NINE: How many symptoms indicate a non-critical crisis?

ANSWER: Five. This is recorded in the third treatise of his (Galen's) *Kitāb al-Buḥrān*. First, ripening. He says: I never saw anyone die who underwent a crisis after ripening. Second, at one time during the crisis, a day of warning should occur which is connected with the strength of the crisis. Third, the nature of the illness. By nature I mean that the fever will become tertian, paroxysmal, ardent, [or change to] pleurisy, or pneumonia. Fourth, demeanor. By demeanor I mean that the patient will be well and at ease or mean and tense. And fifth, the crisis will correspond to the nature of the patient.

QUESTION TEN: How can one recognize a crisis before it occurs?

ANSWER: This is recorded in the third treatise of Galen's *al-Buḥrān*. One looks at the nature of the illness to see whether or not it is caused by the yellow bile, phlegm, or black bile, or a mixture of them. Then **[17b]** look at the periods of the attacks. If they move quickly or periodically, this indicates that the crisis will come quickly. If the periods move slowly and begin at one time and take place all day, this indicates that the crisis will not come until after some time. Then one looks at the ripening. It is one of the strongest symptoms. It is necessary to check the change in the ripening. If a change takes place on a day of warning, this indicates that the departure of the illness from the patient will be on the crisis day, which is connected to that day of warning.

QUESTION ELEVEN: How many symptoms indicate a crisis?

ANSWER: Five. This is recorded in the first treatise of Galen's *Kitāb Ayyām al-buḥrān*, where he says: First, the strongest is the warning that

---

or the better, changed character, or ended by being healed. The end of the disease should witness the elimination of offending humors or excessive matter from the body. This elimination took place on certain definite, or "critical," days of an illness by sweating, purging, urination, or even hemorrhaging so that balance was restored. See Dols, *Medieval Islamic Medicine*, p. 101 n. 13.

precedes it. Second, the scale of the attacks of the fever. Third, the nature of the days [of the crisis]. Fourth, the number of times the crisis occurs. And fifth, when the crisis occurs.[8]

QUESTION TWELVE: On which days is the crisis strong?

ANSWER: This is recorded in Galen's *Ayyām al-buḥrān*, where he says: The strong crisis is on the seventh, the fourteenth, the ninth, the eleventh, and the twentieth and **[18a]** after these the fourth, and after it the third and the eighteenth.[9]

QUESTION THIRTEEN: On which days is the crisis bad and on which days is there no crisis?

ANSWER: This is recorded in Galen's *Ayyām al-buḥrān*. The sixth [is bad]. The twelfth and sixteenth are not crisis days, nor is the ninth.

QUESTION FOURTEEN: What do you say of the days beyond the twentieth?

ANSWER: This is recorded in Galen's *Kitāb Ayyām al-buḥrān*, where he says: As for the twenty-first, it is a day of crisis and likewise the twentieth and twenty-seventh. I noticed that the crisis has the greatest chance of happening on the twenty-eighth. On the thirtieth it is very strong. On the fortieth it is stronger. On the twenty-fourth and thirty-first, the crisis is at its peak, but much less so on the thirty-seventh, so that it could be among the non-crisis or crisis days. As for the rest of the days between the twentieth and fortieth, they are non-crisis days.[10]

QUESTION FIFTEEN: What are the days between the twentieth and fortieth that are crisis **[18b]** and non-crisis days?

ANSWER: The twelfth, twenty-second, twenty-fifth, twenty-sixth, twenty-ninth, thirtieth, thirty-second, thirty-fifth, thirty-sixth, thirty-eighth, and thirty-ninth.[11]

QUESTION: SIXTEEN: What do you say of the days beyond the fortieth?

ANSWER: Galen said: They all show weak activity. The passing of the illness during this time is either a result of ripening or abscesses. It

---

[8] The Arabic of this work ["Book on the Days of Crises"] has not been published: *GAS* III, 96; and Ullmann, *Medizin*, p. 43. For this answer, cf. al-Rāzī, *al-Ḥāwī*, XVIII, 168–70.

[9] Cf. al-Rāzī, *al-Ḥāwī*, XVIII, 16.

[10] Cf. *ibid.*, XVIII, 171.

[11] Cf. *ibid.*

most often happens by vomiting. There can occur a crisis from vomiting during these days, but that is exceedingly rare. I saw that Hippocrates[12] included all of the days after the fortieth except the sixtieth, eightieth, and one hundred and twentieth. Then Galen says: There are some illnesses in which the crisis lasts seven months or seven years.[13]

QUESTION SEVENTEEN: What happens if there is a crisis of the inflamation on the convex side (top) of the liver?

ANSWER: This is recorded in Galen's *Kitāb al-Buḥrān*. One of three things: a nosebleed **[19a]** on the right side, or a favorable amount of perspiration, or a favorable amount of urine. Sometimes two of these things occur and sometimes all of them.

QUESTION EIGHTEEN: What happens if there is a crisis of the inflamation in the cavity (bottom) of the liver?

ANSWER: This is recorded in Galen's *Kitāb al-Buḥrān*, where he says: One of three things: a disparity in the bile, or perspiration, or vomiting.

QUESTION NINETEEN: What is the crisis that resembles tertian fever?

ANSWER: It is [in] the bile, or a disparity [in perspiration] or heavy perspiration all over the body.

QUESTION TWENTY: What is the crisis that resembles paroxysmal fever?

ANSWER: Vomiting a lot of phlegm and heavy perspiration flowing from the entire body.

---

12 On Hippocrates (d. *ca.* 377 BC), see *GAL S* III, index; *GAS* III, 23–47; Ullmann, *Medizin*, pp. 25–35, index; *EI*[2], *Supplement*, *s.v.* "Buḳrāṭ" (A. Dietrich). On this reference to Hippocrates, see his *Hippocratic Writings*, Adams trans., p. 50, where there is no mention of the hundred and twentieth day, but in Chadwick *et al.* trans., p. 101, there is mention of this day.

13 For this entire answer, cf. al-Rāzī, *al-Ḥāwī*, XVIII, 172.

CHAPTER FOUR

FAVORABLE AND DANGEROUS SYMPTOMS, COMPRISING TWENTY QUESTIONS

QUESTION ONE: If a person has a fever accompanied by a dry cough and then the fever diminishes but the cough remains, what does this foretell and why?

ANSWER: This is recorded in the tenth treatise of *al-Malakī*, where the author says: This foretells that abscesses will occur in the joints. This is because the lingering cough indicates that the substance causing the **[19b]** illness remains and has not ripened. The crisis of this substance is frequently indicated by an abscess.[1]

QUESTION TWO: If the white of the eye is red and the veins in it are dark colored or black, what does this indicate and why?

ANSWER: This is recorded in the tenth treatise of *al-Malakī*, where the author says: This indicates certain death. This is because redness of the eye, if it does not come from ophthalmia, indicates that the brain and its covering (membrane) are full of bloody substances. The darkness or blackness of the veins of the eye indicates the coldness of the eye, and this is a particular sign of [impending] death.[2]

QUESTION THREE: If the white of the eye is visible during sleep and is not the patient's normal condition and vomiting does not follow, what does this indicate?

ANSWER: This indicates [impending] death because it indicates a weakness of the brain.[3]

QUESTION FOUR: If an ardent fever is accompanied by a coldness at the extremities and pimples appear on the tongue, what does this indicate?

ANSWER: This is recorded in the tenth treatise of *al-Malakī*, where the author says: This indicates that death is near. The pimples indicate that there are ulcers in the esophagus and stomach.[4]

---

1 *Al-Malakī*, I, 399.

2 *Ibid.*, I, 415.

3 *Ibid.*, I, 416.

4 *Ibid.*

QUESTION FIVE: If the body **[20a]** of a sick person has a chronic ulcer that turns green or black, what does this indicate?

ANSWER: This is recorded in the tenth treatise of *al-Malakī*. This is a bad symptom because, when a patient's condition is terminal, the stricken organ dies before all other organs because of the weakness of the innate heat therein.[5]

QUESTION SIX: If an acute fever occurs and the inside of the body is aflame with thirst while the outside is cold, what does this indicate?

ANSWER: This is recorded in the tenth treatise of *al-Malakī*. This is a sign of death because it indicates a hot inflamation inside the body; the heat is reflected toward the inflamation and the blood flows to it, thus burning the inside of the body.[6]

QUESTION SEVEN: If someone has an acute fever with a high temperature and the temperature abates and the touch of the body is agreeable without cause, what does this indicate?

ANSWER: This indicates that death is near because the heat sinks to the body. It burns the interior while the vital faculty resists it with all of its power in order to repel the substance of the illness. But as it lacks the ability to do so, this faculty declines and the patient dies.[7]

QUESTION EIGHT: How does one determine if **[20b]** the substance [of the illness] is localized in the urinary organs so that it warns that the crisis will occur there?

ANSWER: This is recorded in the *Kulliyyāt al-Qānūn*, where the author says: A heaviness in the bladder, retention of excrement, lack of symptoms of diarrhea, vomiting, nosebleeds, a burning in the urethra, and an aggravation and viscosity of the urine indicate this during this period. There may also be sediment in the urine.[8]

QUESTION NINE: How does one determine if the substance [of the illness] is localized in the bowels so that it warns that the crisis will occur there?

ANSWER: This is recorded in Ibn Sīnā's *al-Qānūn*. A small amount of urine, colic throughout the belly and a residue at the bottom of it, a lack of symptoms of vomiting, the occurrence of a gurgling noise, the

5 *Ibid*.
6 *Ibid*.
7 *Ibid*., I, 416–17.
8 *Al-Qānūn*, III, 84.

inflamation of the ureter, the increase in the color of the excrement, the elevation of the hypochondrium and its protrusion, and the transformation of a gurgle to a pain in the back indicate this. The pulse may be small and strong but not hard. A diarrhea crisis is usually indicated by a small amount of nosebleeding and perspiration and much disparity [in perspiration], especially for someone who usually drinks cold water. It has been said that when the urine, after a crisis over a tertian fever, is colorless and thin, one should expect a disparity (i.e., an extreme soreness) as if [the urethra] is being scraped raw while urinating.[9]

QUESTION TEN: How does one determine if the substance **[21a]** [of the illness] is localized in the veins so that it warns that the crisis will occur there?

ANSWER: This is recorded in Ibn Sīnā's *al-Qānūn*. If the pulse is beating strongly, if one clasps his hand to the patient's skin and dampness occurs under it, if the skin turns red and one finds that the skin becomes hotter than usual and its inflamation and redness are more than before, if the urine turns color and becomes viscous, especially if it changes color on the fourth [day] and thickens on the seventh, one should not expect a crisis of the veins with a looseness of the bowels to be predominant.[10]

QUESTION ELEVEN: How does one determine if the crisis is in the vomiting, so that one can be warned of it before it occurs?

ANSWER: This is recorded in *al-Qānūn*. If there occurs a darkness in the eye and night-blindness (nyctalopia), a bitterness in the mouth, a trembling of the lips, a pain in the cardia, a dribbling of saliva, a palpitation [of the heart], and compression and subsidence in the pulse. This is especially so if the patient is struck after this by a shivering and feels cold in the hypochondrium. Thus, you should conclude that a crisis has occurred in the vomiting, especially if the substance [of the illness] is yellow and the patient has a yellow face.[11]

QUESTION TWELVE: How does one determine if the crisis is in the nosebleed?

ANSWER: If the patient sees **[21b]** red threads, is radiant and has a very shiny and red face, nose and eyes; tears flow all at once; the pulse heightens, is agitated and quickens; the nose itches; the head is extremely hot; and there is a throbbing headache, one should expect a nosebleed.

[9] *Ibid.*

[10] *Ibid.*, III, 83–84.

[11] *Ibid.*, III, 82–83.

This is especially the case if the illness, age, habit, and temperament indicate that the substance [of the illness] is bloody. Moreover, if the substance is yellow, there is a crisis in nosebleed.[12]

QUESTION THIRTEEN: What do you say regarding dropsy that occurs after acute illnesses? If it is accompanied by a fever and pain, what does this indicate?

ANSWER: This is recorded in *al-Malakī.* This is bad, deadly. This is because when dropsy occurs from coldness of the liver and a decline in the [vital] faculty generating the blood, its cure is to apply heat and the use of hot medicines. When we use things like this, we increase the strength of the fever and the pain. If there is pain, it is only caused by a hot inflamation or the burning of the heat [of the fever]. When we use cold things to make the fever subside, we increase the dropsy and that is why the patient dies in most cases.[13]

QUESTION FOURTEEN: If you see someone who suffers from mental confusion and who is fully sensible when he awakens, but if he remains awake **[22a]** for a long time the confusion returns, what does this indicate?

ANSWER: This is recorded in *al-Malakī.* This is a favorable sign because nature overcomes the substance of the illness during the time of sleep and ripens it with its strength. It is necessary to know, however, that a good mental condition is not a good sign in every illness, for people who hemorrhage and have tuberculosis die although they are of sound mind. But this is not so in acute illnesses or illnesses of the head.[14]

QUESTION FIFTEEN: If someone with a cerebral disease sneezes, what does this indicate?

ANSWER: This is recorded in *al-Malakī.* This is a favorable sign because the brain and its interior are able to repel the excess and the harmful thing.[15] Therefore, Galen said in *al-ʿIlal wa-l-aʿrāḍ*:[16] Sneezing, if not from a cold, is one of the most beneficial things for a head filled with steam. On the other hand, it is unfavorable in all other illnesses of the chest because it irritates the chest, and a substance [of an illness] descends to it.

---

12 *Ibid.*, III, 83.

13 *Al-Malakī*, I, 426.

14 *Ibid.*, I, 430. See Dols, *Majnūn*, p. 70.

15 *Al-Malakī*, I, 430.

16 Also called *Kitāb al-ʿIlal wa-l-aʿrāḍ* ["Book on Illnesses and Symptoms"]. The Arabic of this text has not been published: see *GAS* III, 89–90; Ullmann, *Medizin*, p. 42.

QUESTION SIXTEEN: If snakes leave the excrement on one of the crisis days, what does this indicate?

ANSWER: This is recorded in *al-Malakī*. This is a favorable sign because nature is able to repel the harmful substance, and the snakes are repelled together with what is repelled by nature's strength.[17]

[22b] QUESTION SEVENTEEN: If you saw someone suffering from deafness that had occurred immediately after an acute fever and he was then struck by a case of runny diarrhea, what does this indicate?

ANSWER: This deafness results from an ascendance of bile to the head. If that bile descends, the deafness stops. Likewise, if someone suffered from deafness, that disparity [in bile] would stop and in this case we have the opposite condition to what occurred before.[18]

QUESTION: EIGHTEEN: If hemorrhoids appear, on what occasions are they a favorable sign?

ANSWER: The author of *al-Malakī* said: If hemorrhoids occur to people who suffer from melancholia and a cerebral disease, this is a favorable sign because of the descent of the substance [of the illness] from the top [of the body] to the bottom.[19]

QUESTION NINETEEN: If someone with an ardent fever shivers on a crisis day, what does this indicate?

ANSWER: This is recorded in *al-Malakī*. This indicates its termination, because remittent fever comes from the putrid mixture within the arteries and the veins [and goes to the external organs]. The shivering results from the departure of that mixture from the arteries and veins and also from its arrival at the sensory organs.[20]

QUESTION TWENTY: How do you judge the health of someone with pleurisy or pneumonia based on what he spits out?

ANSWER: **[23a]** This is recorded in *al-Malakī*. If what is spit out at the beginning of the illness is thin and colorless and, then, becomes viscous shortly afterwards [and is spit out] with ease and without effort, and one expels it forcefully, and it is not black, green, or yellow, and it does not have an odor, this indicates that the illness has ripened and will last a short time and good health will return.[21]

---

17 *Al-Malakī*, I, 430.
18 *Ibid*.
19 *Ibid*., I, 431.
20 *Ibid*., I, 432.
21 *Ibid*., I, 431.

CHAPTER FIVE

ON SIMPLE DRUGS,[1] COMPRISING TWENTY QUESTIONS

QUESTION ONE: If a mild temperature combines with a fine viscous essence or a medium essence, how will it taste?

ANSWER: This is recorded in the second treatise of Ibn Riḍwān's *al-Uṣūl*,[2] where he says: A mild temperature with a viscous essence causes a sweet taste. A fine essence makes a fatty taste and a medium essence makes a flat taste.

QUESTION TWO: If coldness combines with a fine essence or a viscous essence or a medium essence, how will it taste?

ANSWER: This is recorded in the second treatise of Ibn Riḍwān's *Kitāb al-Uṣūl*. If coldness combines with a viscous essence, an acrid taste will occur. If it combines with a fine essence, a sour taste will occur. And if it combines with a medium essence, an astringent taste will occur.

QUESTION THREE: If a rising temperature combines with a viscous, **[23b]** fine, or medium essence, how will it taste?

ANSWER: This is recorded in Ibn Riḍwān's *Kitāb al-Uṣūl*. If a rising temperature combines with a viscous essence, the taste will be bitter. If a rising temperature combines with a fine essence, the taste will be acrid. If a rising temperature combines with a medium essence, the taste will be salty.

QUESTION FOUR: Into how many classifications are a falling manna[3] divided, how many are there, and from where is each obtained?

---

[1] For a brief introduction to Islamic pharmacology, see *EI*^{2}, *s.v.* "Adwiya" (B. Lewin); and for more details, especially Martin Levey, *Early Arabic Pharmacology: An Introduction Based on Ancient and Medieval Sources* (Leiden: E.J. Brill, 1973).

[2] On Ibn Riḍwān (d. 453/1061), see Joseph Schacht and Max Meyerhof, *The Medico-Philosophical Controversy Between Ibn Butlan of Baghdad and Ibn Ridwan of Cairo*, Faculty of Arts Publication No. 13, the Egyptian University (Cairo, 1937), pp. 1–51; *EI*^{2}, *s.v.* "Ibn Riḍwān" (Schacht); especially Michael Dols, *Medieval Islamic Medicine*, pp. 54–66; Lawrence I. Conrad, "Scholarship and Social Context: A Medical Case from the Eleventh-Century Near East," in Don Bates, ed., *Knowledge and the Scholarly Medical Traditions* (Cambridge: Cambridge University Press, 1995), pp. 84–100. His *Kitāb al-Uṣūl fī l-ṭibb* ["Book on the Principles of Medicine"] only exists in a Hebrew translation: Schacht and Meyerhof, *Controversy*, p. 41.

[3] *Amnān* (pl.), *mann* (s.): al-Samarqandī, p. 220; John Chardin, *Travels in Persia 1673–1677* (repr. New York: Dover, 1988), p. 141.

ANSWER: This is recorded in the eleventh treatise of al-Tamīmī's *al-Murshid*,[4] where he says: As for their classifications, there are two. One is a kind that drops [from the air] on trees. Some have a costive taste like dodder (*kushūth*),[5] some are sharp like dodder (*afthīmūn*),[6] some are sightly bitter and fragrant like Indian, Ethiopian, and Yemeni turmeric,[7] kamala,[8] ladanum,[9] and lac.[10] These are the kinds of aerial medications that fall on trees. As for the second classification of manna, it is sweet essences that dissolve in water and fire, and freeze in cold weather like manna (*taranjubīn*)[11] and honey.[12] As for their number, there are fifteen: honey, sugar of *asclepias gigantea*,[13] manna (*taranjubīn*), honey (*kazankubīn*),[14] —,[15] siracost,[16] manna, wax,[17] ladanum, lac, turmeric, kamala, dodder (*kushūth*), dodder (*afthīmūn*), and sugar. Honey (*'asal*), said al-Tamīmī in **[24a]** his *al-Murshid*, falls from the sky in every country and every region, inhabited and uninhabited. It falls on the leaves of different kinds of flowers and blossoms. As for sugar of *asclepias gigantea*, it is manna that falls on the leaves of the *asclepias gigantea* as moisture like the falling of dew on plants. It acquires from the *asclepias gigantea* an unrestricted force of nature. It congeals on the leaves. As for manna (*taranjubīn*), it is a manna that falls on the thorns of the *shibriq* tree.[18] On

---

[4] Only part of al-Tamīmī's *al-Murshid ilā jawāhir al-aghdhiya wa-quwā l-mufradāt min al-adwiya* ["Guide to the Essences of Nutrition and the Strengths of Simple Drugs"] is extant and has not been published: *GAL* I, 237 and *S* I, 422; *GAS* III, 318; Ullmann, *Medizin*, p. 269.

[5] Al-Samarqandī, pp. 64, 176.

[6] Al-Kindī, pp. 233–34; al-Samarqandī, pp. 64, 176.

[7] *Wars*: Hava, p. 863, calls it *memecylon tinctorium*; Steingass, p. 1463, calls it saffron; *EI*², *s.v.* "Wars" (Penelope C. Johnstone), a yellow dye.

[8] *Qanbīl*: al-Kindī, p. 318; al-Samarqandī, p. 215.

[9] *Lādhan*: al-Kindī, p. 329; al-Samarqandī, pp. 64, 176.

[10] *Lukk*: al-Samarqandī, p. 175.

[11] *Ibid.*, pp. 202, 220.

[12] *'Asal*: al-Kindī, pp. 304; al-Samarqandī, p. 172. See Arabic text.

[13] *Sukkar al-'ushar*: al-Kindī, pp. 284, 304; al-Samarqandī, pp. 174, 203; Maimonides, no. 178 (English trans. Fred Rosner as *Moses Maimonides' Glossary of Drug Names* [Philadelphia: American Philosophical Society, 1979]); Hava, p. 474; and Martin Levey, trans., *Medieval Arabic Toxicology: The Book on Poisons of Ibn al-Waḥshīya and Its Relation to Early Indian and Greek Texts*, in *Transactions of the American Philosophical Society*, New Series, 56.7 (Philadelphia, 1966), p. 122.

[14] Cf. Steingass, p. 1027, *kazāngubīn*.

[15] Word unidentified.

[16] *Shirkhist*: al-Samarqandī, p. 203.

[17] *Sham'*: cf. al-Kindī, p. 294.

[18] Dozy, I, 720; al-Dīnawarī, *Kitāb al-Nabāt*, II, ed. Muḥammad Ḥamīd Allāh (Cairo: Institut Français d'Archéologie Orientale, 1973), pp. 60–61.

this plant is a fruit like the mungo bean.[19] It grows in Khurāsān. As for honey (*kazankubīn*), it is a manna that falls in Khurāsān on the leaves of the tamarisk (*ṭarfā'*) and the tamarisk (*athl*).[20] As for —,[21] it is a manna that falls on the leaves of the Egyptian willow.[22] As for siracost, it is a manna that falls in Herāt on a kind of thorn that has a cold temperature. As for manna itself, it falls on pomegranate[23] blossoms and leaves. It is wild pomegranate.[24] It also falls on the leaves of Christ's thorn,[25] the peach,[26] and the acorn[27] in the Yemen. As for wax, doctors agree with what al-Tamīmī says in his *al-Murshid*. As for myself, I am not of their opinion. Instead, I believe that wax is a substance full of holes made from the saliva of bees and secreted from their stomachs just as silk is made from the saliva of silk worms. The evidence for this is that you can see a change in the color of the wax according to the age of the bees year after year. We see that the wax changes with the age of the bees, and each year a different color is formed. Thus, we find that **[24b]** the wax of the young bees, called *ṭurūd*, is pure white the first year. The second year, it changes to yellow. The third year, the yellow is darker. The fourth year, it becomes red. The fifth year, the red is much darker. The sixth year, it turns black. The seventh year, it is dark black, and this is the last year the bees make it. As for ladanum, it is one of the mannas that falls like dew. It mostly falls on the island of Cyprus on trees on which the sheep of that island graze. If sheep graze on the leaves of this plant and tread on it with their hooves, it becomes suspended from the hair of their whiskers and from their hooves. It accumulates layer upon layer until it becomes like a cake, which is called the moist hyssop,[28] hanging from the tails of the sheep. The ladanum is collected from the hair of these sheep with iron combs. Dioscorides says: It is manna that falls on

---

19 *Māsh*: al-Kindī, pp. 331–32; al-Samarqandī, p. 226.

20 Both of these names for tamarisk are in Hava, pp. 430 and 3 respectively. See al-Dīnawarī, *al-Nabāt*, II, 110–11, also I, 13–20 (ed. Bernard Lewin as *The Book of Plants of Abū Ḥanīfa ad-Dīnawarī* [Uppsala: Lundequistska Bokhandeln, 1953]). Al-Dīnawarī's book has been analyzed by T. Bauer, *Das Pflanzenbuch des Abū Ḥanīfa ad-Dīnawarī: Inhalt, Aufbau, Quellen* (Wiesbaden: Harrassowitz, 1988).

21 Word unidentified.

22 *Khilāf*: al-Samarqandī, pp. 227–28.

23 *Jullinār al-maẓẓ*: al-Kindī, pp. 253–54; al-Dīnawarī, *al-Nabāt*, II, 275–76.

24 *Rummān*: al-Samarqandī, pp. 176–77.

25 *Sidr*: *ibid.*, p. 221.

26 *Khawkh*: *ibid.*, pp. 29, 215.

27 *Bullūṭ*: al-Kindī, pp. 245–46; al-Samarqandī, p. 211.

28 *Zūfā*: al-Kindī, p. 277; al-Samarqandī, p. 182.

a type of tree called ivy (*qusūs*).[29] If sheep graze on it, it clings to their whiskers and hooves because it is sticky by nature.[30] As for lac, some say it is gum Arabic (resin),[31] but that is not true. The evidence for this is that it is a manna that we find coated on the stalks of the vine from which come the [grape] leaves and grapes. We find the piece of wood on which the lac is present is as thick as the little finger or much smaller. And we find that the lac found on it is many times thicker than the stalk that is carrying it until it is as thick as the thumb or thicker. There is no resinous pliability in the stalks of the vine, **[25a]** although this thin piece of wood is syrupy and coated by it. This indicates that this is a fine aerial substance that falls on the outside of the stalks. They attach to it the property that is instilled in them. It is peculiar to two places in India. One of them is Daybul[32] and the other is al-Ṣamra (?)[33] or Sandān.[34] As for turmeric, it is called saffron[35] and ambergris (*qindīd*)[36] and by others Ethiopian turmeric, but it does not grow in Ethiopia at all. Instead, it can fall in China. It is imported from China to India and called Indian turmeric. It can also fall in the Yemen. There are three kinds. The first falls in China and is imported to India. The second is Ethiopian. It falls in Ethiopia and is imported to Mecca. The third is Yemeni. It falls in the valleys of the Yemen and is imported from there. It falls on a kind of tree resembling mountain balm[37] and in both leaves and flowers. As for kamala, it is one of the falling mannas. It falls in the valleys of the Yemen like the turmeric. As for dodder (*kushūth*), it falls in Iraq and on

---

29 Hava, p. 604.

30 See Robert T. Gunther, trans., *The Greek Herbal of Dioscorides* (1934; repr. New York: Hafner Publishing Co., 1959), p. 68. The ivy is called here *gum cistus*. For the Arabic text, cf. César E. Dubler, *La ‚Materia Médica' de Dioscorides* (Barcelona: Tipografia Emporium, 1953–59), II, 91. On Dioscorides (d. 1st cent. BC), see *GAL* I, 206–207 and *S* I, 369–71; *GAS* III, 58–60; *EI* ², *s.v.* "Diyusḳuridīs" (Dubler); Ullmann, *Medizin*, pp. 257–63; M.M. Sadek, *The Arabic Materia Medica of Dioscorides* (Quebec: Les Editions du Sphinx, 1983); John M. Riddle, *Dioscorides on Pharmacy and Medicine* (Austin, Texas: University of Texas Press, 1985).

31 *Ṣamgh*: al-Samarqandī, p. 222; *EI* ², *s.v.* "Ṣamgh" (Dietrich).

32 *EI* ², *s.v.* "Daybul" (A.S. Bazmee Ansari).

33 Perhaps Ṣaymūr on the west coast of India. See Yāqūt, *Muʿjam al-buldān*, ed. F. Wüstenfeld (Leipzig: F.A. Brockhaus, 1866–73), III, 444.

34 On the west coast of India north of Ṣaymūr; *ibid.*, III, 165–66.

35 *Ḥuṣṣ*: Steingass, p. 421; Hava, p. 126.

36 Steingass, p. 991; Hava, p. 629; Chardin, *Travels in Persia*, pp. 153–54.

37 *Bādhrūj*: al-Samarqandī, pp. 181–82; Steingass, p. 141. Cf. Levey, *Toxicology*, p. 116.

everything resembling mountain balm. It is purslane.[38] As for dodder (*afthīmūn*), it is one of the mannas that falls from the sky. It falls on a kind of wild thyme called thyme-like (*ṣaʿtīra*). There are three kinds from three countries. The best comes from the island of Crete and comes via Jerusalem or the villages of Palestine. As for sugar, some people are of the opinion that it is one of the mannas that falls from the sky, but it is one of the juices formed by congealing.

[25b] QUESTION FIVE: How many kinds of bitumen are extracted from inside the earth?

ANSWER: Eight kinds. This is recorded in the eleventh treatise of al-Tamīmī's *al-Murshid*. They are ambergris (*ʿanbar*),[39] sandarach,[40] Persian pissasphalt,[41] Maghribi pissasphalt, Jews' bitumen,[42] Iraqi tar,[43] naphtha,[44] and sulphur.[45]

QUESTION SIX: What do you say regarding the fruit of the tamarisk (*ṭarfāʾ*)? Does anyone mention that it is useful for leprosy[46] and if so how does it work?

ANSWER: This is recorded in Ibn Wāfid's *al-Adwiya al-mufrada*,[47] where he says: I have been told on good account that a certain woman got leprosy. She was made to drink several times a mash composed of the roots of the tamarisk and raisins and she was cured. He (Ibn Wāfid) tried it again and it worked. Ibn Wāfid said: I say it works because this illness

---

38 *Ḥawk*: Steingass, p. 434; Hava, p. 150; Kazimirski, I, 516.

39 Al-Kindī, p. 307; al-Samarqandī, pp. 189–90; *EI* 2, *s.v.* "ʿAnbar" (J. Ruska/M. Plessner).

40 *Sandarūs*: al-Kindī, p. 287; al-Samarqandī, p. 236.

41 *Mūmyā fārisī*: Steingass, p. 1349; Hava, p. 740. Cf. *EI* 2, *s.v.* "Mūmiyāʾ" (Dietrich).

42 *Qafr al-yahūd*: Steingass, p. 981; Hava, p. 620.

43 *Qār ʿirāqī*: Steingass, p. 946; Hava, p. 633.

44 *Nafṭ*: al-Samarqandī, p. 227. Cf. *EI* 2, *s.v.* "Nafṭ" (M.E.J. Richards *et al.*).

45 *Kibrīt*: al-Kindī, pp. 322–23; al-Samarqandī, p. 241; *EI* 2, *s.v.* "Kibrīt" (Ullmann).

46 On leprosy, see *EI* 2, *Supplement*, *s.v.* "Djudhām" (Dols); Dols, "Leprosy in Medieval Arabic Medicine," *JHMAS*, 34 (1979), 162–89; *idem*, "The Leper in Medieval Islamic Society," *Speculum*, 58 (1983), 891–916.

47 On Abū l-Mutarrif ʿAbd al-Raḥmān ibn Muḥammad ibn Wāfid al-Lakhmī (d. 467/1074) and his *Kitāb fī l-adwiya al-mufrada* ["Book on Simple Drugs"], see *GAL* I, 485 and *S* I, 887; *EI* 2, *s.v.* "Ibn Wāfid" (J.F.P. Hopkins); Ullmann, *Medizin*, pp. 210, 273, 306; Martin Levey, *Early Arabic Pharmacology*, pp. 111–13, 149. Ibn Wāfid's book has been edited and translated into Spanish by Luisa Fernanda Aguirre de Cárcer as *Kitāb al-Adwiya al-mufrada* (Madrid: Consejo Superior de Investigaciones Científicas Agencia Española de Cooperación Internacional, 1995), I (Spanish trans.) and II (Arabic text). There is a Catalan translation of Ibn Wāfid's book edited by L. Faraudo de Saint-Germian as *El "Libre de les medicines particulars"* (Barcelona, 1943).

in people originates from an inflamation of the spleen or its obstruction. Either of these prevents the drawing of the black bile from the blood and purifying it. This is the reason for the appearance of the disease that they have. When the inflamation goes down, [or] the obstruction is opened because they use this medicine that cuts and removes by nature, they return to health.[48]

QUESTION SEVEN: What do you say regarding the little stones generated in the bladders of people? Is it mentioned if they are of benefit or not for any sickness?

ANSWER: This is recorded in the twelfth treatise of al-Tamīmī's *al-Murshid*, where he says: If the stones generated in the bladder are pulverized and daubed on an eye with leucoma, they will clear it up and forcefully eliminate it.

[26a] QUESTION EIGHT: What is the disease for which a person drinks his own urine and benefits from it?

ANSWER: This is recorded in Ibn Wāfid's *al-Adwiya al-mufrada*, where he says: If a person drinks his own urine, it is of use against the bite of the viper, deadly drugs, and the onset of dropsy.[49]

QUESTION NINE: What is mentioned to be an unusual advantage of ghee[50] and how is this so?

ANSWER: This is recorded in al-Tamīmī's *al-Murshid*, where he says: One of the peculiarities of ghee is that it arrests the illness called leontiasis, which is leprosy. It should be boiled and poured into a wide washbowl or pot and left until it is possible to sit in it. Then the one with this illness sits in it up to his neck. It is continuously poured on his head until it cools. Then he gets out, washes in hot water, and puts on his clothes. If he sticks to this regime for a week, he will be free of this illness for a whole year and it will not increase. But the following year he must repeat this regime.

QUESTION TEN: What is mentioned concerning the benefits of dog milk?

ANSWER: This is recorded in al-Tamīmī's *al-Murshid*, where he says: If the milk of a young dog is daubed on the place of excess hair under

---

48 Ibn Wāfid, pp. 85–86 (Arabic) and pp. 137–37 (Spanish).

49 I was not able to find a reference to this in Ibn Wāfid. He mentions a number of antidotes for the bite of the viper, for example, pp. (Arabic) 87, 99, 138, 173 (and deadly drugs) -74, 190, 210.

50 *Samn*: al-Kindī, p. 286.

the eyelid and then daubed on hair in other places, that hair will never return. This is the case for the rest of the body after it has been plucked. If it is daubed on the places where the teeth of children **[26b]** grow and on their swollen gums when their teeth erupt, the pain subsides and the teeth of the children quickly erupt without pain. It will expel the dead fetus if a woman is pregnant with one.

QUESTION ELEVEN: What is the benefit ascribed to the cores of olive pits and their gum?

ANSWER: This is recorded in al-Tamīmī's *al-Murshid*, where he says: As for the cores inside olive pits, if they are pulverized and mixed with grease and flour and a dressing is made from this, it takes away the whiteness occurring in the nails. As for their gum, Ḥubaysh[51] said: If it is pulverized and copiously applied to a wound, it will heal it.

QUESTION TWELVE: How many hot and dry medicines in the first degree are mentioned by Ibn Wāfid, and what are they?[52]

ANSWER: This is recorded in Ibn Wāfid's *Kitāb al-Adwiya al-mufrada*.[53] As for their number, it is sixty-two. They are wormwood (*afsintīn*),[54] rice, sarcocolla,[55] spong,[56] lavender,[57] melilot,[58] lemon grass,[59] lesser

[51] On Ḥubaysh ibn al-Ḥasan al-A'sam al-Dimashqī (d. end of 3rd/9th cent.), see *GAL* I, 207 and *S* I, 369; *GAS* III, 265–66; Dietrich, *Medicinalia*, pp. 39–42; Ullmann, *Medizin*, p. 119, index; Dodge, *Fihrist*, II, 699.

[52] In the Galenic system, every drug taken from the three realms of nature was categorized by degree as hot, dry, cold, or moist. Therapy was based on the principle of contraries. "Hot" diseases were cured by "cold" remedies, and so forth. See Bürgel, "Medieval Arabic Medicine," pp. 47–48.

[53] The lists of material medica from Ibn Wāfid for the answers to the remaining questions in this section are somewhat problematic. The names of most of these items were not Arabic and therefore were generally not familiar to copyists. Furthermore, many of these names could be spelled in more than one way. The published version of Ibn Wāfid's book can help control the text, but it is based on late and disparate manuscripts. No complete Arabic text of the work has survived. See vol. I (Spanish), 27–31.

[54] Al-Kindī, p. 233; al-Samarqandī, p. 213; *EI*^{2}, *s.v.* "Afsantīn" (L. Kopf).

[55] *Anzarūt*: al-Kindī, p. 236; al-Samarqandī, p. 213, where it is spelled *'anzarūt*; *EI*^{2}, *Supplement*, *s.v.* "Anzarūt" (Dietrich).

[56] *Isfanj*: al-Samarqandī, p. 227.

[57] *Usṭūkhūdūs*: *ibid.*, pp. 187–88.

[58] *Iklīl al-malik*: al-Kindī, p. 235; al-Samarqandī, p. 204; *EI*^{2}, *Supplement*, *s.v.* "Iklīl al-Malik" (Dietrich).

[59] *Idhkhir*: al-Kindī, pp. 225–26; al-Samarqandī, p. 175.

cardamom,[60] flax seed,[61] camomile,[62] mountain balm (*bādranjūya*),[63] Judas tree,[64] oats (*dūsar*),[65] spikenard,[66] agallochum,[67] *ḥarīr*,[68] semolina,[69] white popular,[70] tamarisk (*ṭarfā'*), cabbage,[71] bitter vetch,[72] coriander,[73] grape vine and grapes,[74] dodder (*kushūth*), *kulābī*,[75] ivy (*lablāb*),[76] ladanum, dragonwort,[77] mahlab,[78] manna, storax,[79] indigo,[80] sawdust,[81] chaste tree,[82] ironwood tree,[83] **[27a]** sugar, nard,[84] malabathrum,[85] *sukk*,[86] cypress,[87] laurel (*sarkhas*),[88] sandarach, senna,[89]

---

60 *Abil*: Steingass, p. 10.

61 *Bizr kattān*: al-Samarqandī, p. 193.

62 *Bābūnaj*: al-Kindī, p. 239; *EI* 2, *Supplement*, *s.v.* "Bābūnadj" (Dietrich).

63 Al-Samarqandī, pp. 181–82; and cf. *EI* 2, *s.v.* "Turundjān" (Penelope C. Johnstone).

64 *Dādhī*: al-Kindī, p. 265.

65 Steingass, p. 544.

66 *Dār shīshī'ān*: Steingass, p. 496. Cf. Levey, *Toxicology*, p. 119.

67 *Harnuwwa*: Steingass, p. 1497; Levey, *Toxicology*, p. 127.

68 Al-Kindī, p. 258, and Steingass, p. 418, both call it a flour mixed with milk and oil.

69 *Ḥinṭa*: al-Samarqandī, p. 210.

70 *Ḥawar*: al-Kindī, pp. 262; al-Dīnawarī, *al-Nabāt*, I, 118; *Tuḥfa*, pp. 86–87.

71 *Kurunb*: al-Kindī, p. 326; al-Samarqandī, p. 204.

72 *Karsana*: al-Kindī, p. 324; al-Samarqandī, p. 219.

73 *Kuzbara*: al-Kindī, p. 326; al-Samarqandī, p. 184.

74 *Karm wa-'inab*: al-Kindī, pp. 306–307, 326; al-Samarqandī, p. 225; *EI* 2, *s.v.* "Karm" (L. Bolens and Cl. Cahen).

75 Unidentified.

76 Al-Samarqandī, p. 204.

77 *Lūf*: al-Kindī, p. 331.

78 *Maḥlab*: Steingass, p. 1189, a kind of grain resembling cherry-stones growing in Azerbaijan; Hava, p. 138, *prunus mahaleb*; Levey, *Toxicology*, p. 126.

79 *May'a*: al-Kindī, p. 338; al-Samarqandī, p. 229.

80 *Nīlanj* or *nīlaj*: al-Dīnawarī, *al-Nabāt*, II, 143; Maimonides, nos. 126, 249; *EI* 2, *s.v.* "Nīl" (Dietrich).

81 *Nushāra*: Steingass, p. 1402, rotten wood falling to powder (sawdust).

82 *Banjakusht*: al-Kindī, p. 247; al-Samarqandī, p. 175. This and the previous item are probably one compound, i.e., powder of the chaste tree.

83 *Nārmushk*: al-Samarqandī, p. 195.

84 *Sunbul*: al-Kindī, pp. 286–87; al-Samarqandī, p. 189.

85 *Sādaj*: al-Kindī, p. 279; al-Samarqandī, p. 194.

86 Al-Samarqandī, pp. 159, 197.

87 *Sarw*: al-Kindī, pp. 281–82; al-Samarqandī, p. 224.

88 Steingass, p. 672. Hava, p. 317, gives *sirkhis* as fern.

89 *Sanā*: al-Kindī, p. 286; al-Samarqandī, p. 186.

pistachio,[90] madder,[91] tinder of *fāwaniyā* wood,[92] pine,[93] saltwort,[94] cotton,[95] vetch,[96] kamala, fresh dates, tare,[97] anemone,[98] bush basil,[99] narcissus,[100] spelt,[101] marshmallow,[102] agrimony,[103] agaric,[104] cardamom,[105] and lupine.[106]

QUESTION THIRTEEN: How many hot and moist medicines in the first degree does Ibn Wāfid mention in his book?

ANSWER: Thirteen. They are walnuts,[107] *ḥindim*,[108] chickpeas,[109] beans (*lūbiyā*),[110] almonds,[111] borage,[112] mauve,[113] sesame,[114] jujubes,[115] sugarcane,[116] secacul,[117] satyrion,[118] and orchis (*khuṣā l-kalb*).[119]

---

90 *Fustuq*: al-Samarqandī, pp. 180, 220.

91 *Fūwwa*: *ibid.*, p. 199.

92 *Fāwaniyā qaw*: Steingass, pp. 905.

93 *Ṣanawbar*: al-Kindī, pp. 299–300.

94 *Qāqullā*: Steingass, p. 948; Hava, p. 621.

95 *Quṭn*: al-Kindī, p. 317; al-Samarqandī, p. 219; *EI* 2, *s.v.* "Ḳuṭn" (E. Ashtor *et al.*).

96 *Qilt*: Steingass, p. 984.

97 *Shayyalam* or *shaylam*: al-Dīnawarī, *al-Nabāt*, I, 79–80; *Tuḥfa*, p. 190; Steingass, p. 777.

98 *Shaqā'iq*: al-Samarqandī, p. 236; *EI* 2, *s.v.* "Shaḳā'iḳ al-Nu'mān" (Dietrich).

99 *Shāhisfaram*: al-Kindī, pp. 290–91.

100 *Narjis*: al-Samarqandī, p. 209; *EI* 2, *s.v.* "Nardjis" (Ed.).

101 *Khandarūs*: Maimonides, no. 389.

102 *Khiṭmī*: al-Samarqandī, p. 182.

103 *Ghāfit*: al-Kindī, pp. 309–10; al-Samarqandī, pp. 173–74.

104 *Ghārīqūn*: al-Kindī, p. 309; al-Samarqandī, p. 186.

105 *Qāqulla*: al-Kindī, pp. 313–14; al-Samarqandī, pp. 179, 197.

106 *Turmus*: al-Kindī, pp. 249–50; al-Samarqandī, pp. 29, 225. For this answer, cf. Ibn Wāfid, pp. 19–20 (Arabic) and p. 57 (Spanish).

107 *Jawz*: al-Kindī, pp. 255–56; *EI* 2, *Supplement*, *s.v.* "Djawz" (Dietrich).

108 Al-Dīnawarī calls it a tree with red roots; *al-Nabāt*, I, 140.

109 *Ḥimmiṣ*: al-Kindī, pp. 260–61.

110 *Ibid.*, p. 331.

111 *Lawz*: al-Samarqandī, p. 192.

112 *Lisān thawr*: *ibid.*, p. 181; al-Dīnawarī, *al-Nabāt*, II, 257.

113 *Mulūkh*: al-Samarqandī, pp. 217, 240–41.

114 *Simsim*: al-Kindī, pp. 285–86; *EI* 2, *s.v.* "Simsim" (Dietrich).

115 *'Unnāb*: al-Samarqandī, p. 201; *EI* 2, " 'Unnāb" (A. Dietrich).

116 *Qaṣab*: al-Samarqandī, p. 222. Cf. al-Kindī, p. 316, where it is called false acorus; and *EI* 2, *s.v.* "Ḳaṣab al-Sukkar" (M. Canard and P. Berthier).

117 *Shaqāqul*: al-Kindī, p. 294; al-Samarqandī, pp. 239–40.

118 *Khuṣā l-tha'lab*: *Tuḥfa*, p. 179; Hava, p. 171.

119 *Tuḥfa*, pp. 179–80; Hava, p. 171. For this answer, cf. Ibn Wāfid, p. 20 (Arabic) and p. 57 (Spanish).

QUESTION FOURTEEN: How many cold and dry medicines in the first degree are there?

ANSWER: This is recorded in Ibn Wāfid's *Kitāb al-Adwiya al-mufrada*. Forty-four, although they are forty-five. They are myrtle,[120] lichen,[121] acacia (*aqāqiyā*),[122] emblic myrobalan (*amlaj*),[123] michaelmas daisy,[124] beans (*bāqillā*),[125] acorns, white thorn,[126] coral,[127] papyrus,[128] common millet,[129] diss,[130] pearl millet (*dukhn*),[131] elm,[132] teazel,[133] myrobalan (*halīlaj*),[134] rose,[135] azerole,[136] henna,[137] **[27b]** sorrel,[138] water caltrop,[139] liverwort,[140] pear,[141] salsify,[142] mungo bean, false bdellium,[143] date palm,[144] Christ's thorn, *sādarwān*,[145] thin husked barley,[146]

---

120 *Āss*: al-Samarqandī, pp. 177–78; *EI* 2, *Supplement*, *s.v.* "Ās" (Dietrich).

121 *Ushna*: al-Kindī, p. 232; al-Samarqandī, pp. 194, 209.

122 Al-Kindī, p. 234; al-Samarqandī, p. 211.

123 Al-Kindī, p. 235; al-Samarqandī, pp. 26, 185.

124 *Asṭūr aṭīqūs*: Gunther, *Dioscorides*, pp. 510–11; Dubler, *Materia Médica*, II, 352; Dozy, I, 21, aster atticus, *asṭūr aṭīqūs*.

125 Al-Kindī, pp. 240–41; al-Samarqandī, p. 241.

126 *Bādhāward*: Steingass, p. 141.

127 *Basad*: al-Kindī, pp. 243–44; al-Samarqandī, pp. 185, 221.

128 *Bardī*: Maimonides, no. 46; *Tuḥfa*, p. 39.

129 *Jāwars*: al-Samarqandī, pp. 213, 223; *EI* 2, *Supplement*, *s.v.* "Djāwars" (Dietrich).

130 *Dīs*: Wehr, p. 305.

131 *Ibid*., p. 275. Steingass, p. 505, and Hava, p. 199, both say just millet.

132 *Dardār*: Steingass, p. 511; Hava, p. 200; Wehr, p. 277.

133 *Dibsāqūs*: Gunther, *Dioscorides*, p. 244; Dubler, *Materia Médica*, II, 244.

134 Al-Kindī, p. 342; al-Samarqandī, pp. 26, 184; *EI* 2, *Supplement*, *s.v.* "Halīladj" (Dietrich).

135 *Ward*: al-Kindī, pp. 344–45; al-Samarqandī, p. 220; *EI* 2, *s.v.* "Ward" (Penelope C. Johnstone).

136 *Za'rūr*: al-Samarqandī, p. 179; Hava, p. 289.

137 *Ḥinnā'*: al-Kindī, pp. 261–62; al-Samarqandī, p. 191; *EI* 2, *s.v.* "Ḥinnā'" (G.S. Colin).

138 *Ḥummād*: al-Samarqandī, pp. 205, 220; Hava, p. 143.

139 *Ḥasak*: al-Kindī, p. 259; al-Samarqandī, p. 204.

140 *Ḥazāz al-sakhr*: Maimonides, no. 152; Hava, p. 121.

141 *Kumathrā*: al-Samarqandī, pp. 177, 222.

142 *Liḥyat al-tays*: Steingass, p. 1119; Hava, p. 682; Levey, *Toxicology*, p. 125.

143 *Muql*: al-Kindī, p. 336; al-Samarqandī, p. 185.

144 *Nakhla*: Steingass, p. 1392; *EI* 2, *s.v.* "Nakhl" (F. Viré).

145 Al-Kindī, pp. 278–79; *Tuḥfa*, pp. 161–62.

146 *Sult*: Hava, p. 330; R.B. Serjeant, "The Cultivation of Cereals in Mediaeval Yemen," *Arabian Studies* 1 (1974), 44–45.

'alas wheat,[147] lesser bindweed,[148] oats (*qurṭumān*),[149] arbutus,[150] sugar-cane, pomegranate, cotton-thistle,[151] barley,[152] mulberry,[153] apples,[154] quince,[155] vinegar, carob,[156] Egyptian willow, and isinglass.[157]

QUESTION FIFTEEN: How many cold and moist medicines in the first degree does Ibn Wāfid mention in his simples (*mufradāt*)?

ANSWER: Eleven. They are plums,[158] spinach,[159] plane tree,[160] violet,[161] endive,[162] water lily,[163] small black plums,[164] atriplex,[165] licorice,[166] beets,[167] and mallow.[168]

QUESTION SIXTEEN: How many hot and dry medicines in the second degree does Ibn Wāfid mention?

ANSWER: Sixty-one (*sic*). They are nettles,[169] ungues (odorati),[170]

---

147 Hava, p. 494; Lane, *Lexicon*, I.5, 2130; Serjeant, "Cereals," pp. 43–44.

148 *'Ullayq*: cf. Wehr, p. 634; Hava, p. 495, who also has *'alīq*, barley. Steingass, p. 865, has barley and dodder.

149 Hava, p. 599. Cf. Steingass, p. 964, who has tares.

150 *Qātil abī-hi*: Maimonides, no. 328.

151 *Shukā'ā*: Dozy, I, 778; Kazimirski, I, 1259; *EI* 2, *s.v.* "Shukā'ā" (Dietrich). Cf. Hava, p. 373, *shukā'ī*.

152 *Sha'īr*: al-Kindī, p. 293; al-Samarqandī, p. 196; *EI* 2, *s.v.* "Sha'īr" (D. Waines).

153 *Tūt*: Lane, *Lexicon*, I.1, 321; *EI* 2, *s.v.* "Tūt" (Penelope C. Johnstone).

154 *EI* 2, *s.v.* "Tuffāḥ" (A. Dietrich).

155 *Safarjal*: al-Kindī, pp. 282–83; al-Samarqandī, p. 176.

156 *Kharnūb*: al-Samarqandī, p. 239.

157 *Ghirā'*: Hava, p. 523; Steingass, p. 882, who calls it an aromatic plant. For this answer, cf. Ibn Wāfid, p. 20 (Arabic) and p. 58 (Spanish).

158 *Ijjāṣ*: al-Kindī, p. 225; al-Samarqandī, pp. 177, 203.

159 *Isfānākh*: al-Samarqandī, p. 216.

160 *Dulb*: Steingass, p. 531; Hava, p. 213; Levey, *Toxicology*, p. 119.

161 *Banafsaj*: al-Kindī, p. 247.

162 *Hundabā'*: *ibid.*, pp. 342–43; al-Samarqandī, p. 173; *EI* 2, *Supplement*, *s.v.* "Hindibā'" (Dietrich).

163 *Nūfar*: Steingass, p. 1435.

164 *Qarāsiyā*: cf. Hava, p. 598, and Wehr, p. 756, both of whom call it *qarāsiyya*. Steingass, p. 961, calls it a cherry.

165 *Qaṭaf*: Dozy, II, 376; Kazimirski, II, 772–73. Cf. Steingass, p. 978.

166 *Sūs*: al-Kindī, pp. 288–89; *EI* 2, *s.v.* "Sūs" (O. Kahl).

167 *Silq*: al-Kindī, pp. 284–85; al-Samarqandī, p. 204.

168 *Khubbāzā*: al-Samarqandī, p. 198, *khubbāzī*; Hava, p. 155. For this answer, cf. Ibn Wāfid, p. 20 (Arabic) and p. 58 (Spanish).

169 *Anjura*: Steingass, p. 106; Hava, p. 751.

170 *Aẓfār*: cf. Hava, p. 446; Levey, *Toxicology*, p. 115.

ebony,[171] —,[172] the herb pimpernel,[173] sage,[174] common calamint,[175] mountain balm, pepper,[176] terebinth of balsam,[177] nutmeg (*jawz bawwa*),[178] walnuts, hazelnuts,[179] nux vomica,[180] germander (*ja'da*),[181] carrots,[182] birdlime,[183] dirt from clay beehives,[184] turmeric, Aristolochia,[185] wild ginger (*zurunbād*),[186] saffron (*za'farān*),[187] fenugreek,[188] sweet basil,[189] jasmine,[190] Jews' bitumen, castoreum,[191] **[28a]** frankincense,[192] the herb gound-pine,[193] the herb germander (*kamādaryūs*),[194] lukk, *meum athamanticum*,[195] mastix,[196] garum,[197] musk,[198] nascaptha,[199] eglantine,[200] narcissus, lily,[201] turnips,[202] sweet cyperus,[203]

---

171 *Abnūs*: *Tuḥfa*, p. 14; *EI*², *Supplement*, *s.v.* "Abanūs" (J. Hell).

172 Word unidentified, see Arabic text.

173 *Anāghulus*: Steingass, p. 103; *anāghālīs* in Maimonides, no. 16.

174 *Asfāqus*: *Tuḥfa*, p. 17.

175 *Faranjmushk*: S. Haim, *New Persian-English Dictionary* (Tehran: Beroukhim, 1960), II, 474. Steingass, p. 922, calls it sweet basil.

176 *Bahār*: Steingass, p. 209; Hava, p. 49.

177 *Buṭm balasān*: cf. al-Kindī, p. 245; al-Samarqandī, pp. 228, 230.

178 Al-Kindī, p. 250; al-Samarqandī, p. 229.

179 *Jillawz*: Steingass, p. 369; Hava, p. 95.

180 *Jawz al-raqa'*: al-Samarqandī, p. 218.

181 Steingass, p. 364; Levey, *Toxicology*, p. 117.

182 *Jazar*: al-Kindī, pp. 252–53. Cf. al-Samarqandī, p. 217.

183 *Dibq*: Steingass, p. 503; Hava, p. 196, who also says mistletoe.

184 *Wasakh al-kawā'ir*: Hava, p. 669.

185 *Zarāwand*: al-Kindī, p. 273; al-Samarqandī, p. 193.

186 Al-Kindī, p. 274.

187 *Ibid.*, pp. 275–76; al-Samarqandī, p. 180; *EI*², *s.v.* "Za'farān" as medicament (F. Sanagustin).

188 *Ḥulba*: al-Kindī, pp. 259–60.

189 *Ḥamāḥim*: *Tuḥfa*, p. 81; Steingass, pp. 430, 185; Hava, p. 141.

190 *Yāsamīn*: al-Samarqandī, p. 228; *EI*², *s.v.* "Yāsāmīn" (Viré).

191 *Jundbīdastar*: al-Kindī, p. 254; al-Samarqandī, p. 171.

192 *Kundur*: al-Kindī, p. 328; al-Samarqandī, p. 188.

193 *Kamāfīṭus*: *Tuḥfa*, pp. 97–98; Steingass, p. 1047.

194 *Tuḥfa*, p. 98; Steingass, p. 1046.

195 *Mū* or *muww*: Ibn Wāfid, p. 413 (Spanish).

196 *Maṣṭakī*: al-Samarqandī, p. 179; and Steingass, p. 1253, both have *maṣṭakā*.

197 *Murrī*: al-Samarqandī, pp. 206–207, 238.

198 *Misk*: *ibid.*, p. 193; Chardin, *Travels in Persia*, pp. 150–52; *EI*², *s.v.* "Misk" (Dietrich).

199 *Bunk*: Steingass, p. 203; Hava, p. 47.

200 *Nisrīn*: al-Samarqandī, p. 230.

201 *Sūsan*: al-Kindī, p. 289; al-Samarqandī, pp. 182, 209; *EI*², *s.v.* "Sūsan" (Penelope C. Johnstone).

202 *Saljam*: *Tuḥfa*, pp. 163–64; Hava, p. 330; Levey, *Toxicology*, p. 121; Wehr, p. 420.

scolopender,[204] colchicum,[205] honey, ambergris (*'anbar*), aloe (*'ūd*),[206] wild leek,[207] *falanja*,[208] *fāghara*,[209] aloe (*ṣabr*),[210] carthamus,[211] taro,[212] squirting cucumber,[213] false Acorus,[214] rhubarb,[215] hemp,[216] figs,[217] yellow gillyflower,[218] asphodel,[219] and castor oil plant.[220]

QUESTION SEVENTEEN: How many hot and moist medicines in the second degree does Ibn Wāfid mention?

ANSWER: Six. They are behen,[221] rocket,[222] cassa tora,[223] honeywort,[224] *mughāth*,[225] and coconuts.[226]

QUESTION EIGHTEEN: How many cold and dry medicines in the second degree does Ibn Wāfid mention?

ANSWER: Thirteen. They are berberis,[227] fleawort seeds,[228] pome-

---

203 *Sa'd*: al-Kindī, p. 282; al-Samarqandī, p. 189.

204 *Saqūlūfandūriyyūn*: *Tuḥfa*, p. 172; Dozy, I, 664. In the Vienna manuscript this word is divided in two and given as two different substances.

205 *Sūranjān*: al-Kindī, pp. 287–88; al-Samarqandī, pp. 190, 223.

206 Cf. al-Kindī, pp. 307–308; Hava, pp. 507–508; Levey, *Toxicology*, p. 123.

207 *Farāsīyūn*: *Tuḥfa*, p. 143, *marrube* in French.

208 A red seed used as a perfume; Steingass, p. 938.

209 A spice the size of a vetch; *ibid.*, p. 904. Hava, p. 569, calls it lotus of India and cubeb.

210 Al-Kindī, p. 297; al-Samarqandī, p. 198; *EI* [2], *s.v.* "Ṣabr" (Dietrich).

211 *Qirṭim*: al-Samarqandī, p. 193.

212 *Qulqās*: *Tuḥfa*, pp. 106–107, 170; Steingass, p. 985; Hava, p. 625; Wehr, p. 787.

213 *Qiththā' al-ḥimār*: Maimonides, no. 292; Hava, p. 588. Cf. *Tuḥfa*, pp. 151–52.

214 *Qaṣab al-dharīra*: al-Kindī, p. 316; Levey, *Toxicology*, p. 124.

215 *Rāwand*: al-Samarqandī, p. 174; *Tuḥfa*, pp. 156–57.

216 *Shahdānaj*: al-Samarqandī, pp. 205–206; *EI* [2], *s.v.* "Shahdānadj" (F. Rosenthal).

217 *Tīn*: al-Kindī, p. 250; *EI* [2], *s.v.* "Tīn" (D. Waines).

218 *Khīrī*: al-Samarqandī, p. 230.

219 *Khunthā*: *Tuḥfa*, p. 180.

220 *Khirwa'*: al-Kindī, p. 264; al-Samarqandī, p. 206. For this answer, cf. Ibn Wāfid, p. 21 (Arabic) and pp. 58–59 (Spanish).

221 *Bahman*: *Tuḥfa*, p. 33; Dozy, I, 123; Steingass, p. 212.

222 *Jirjīr*: al-Kindī, p. 252.

223 *Ḥabb al-qilqil*: al-Dīnawarī, *al-Nabāt*, II, 223–24; *Tuḥfa*, pp. 81, 147.

224 *Lisān al-'uṣfūr*: Dozy, II, 529; Steingass, p. 1121.

225 *Mughāth*: al-Dīnawarī, *al-Nabāt*, II, 912; *Tuḥfa*, p. 122, *glossostamon brugieri*.

226 *Nārajīl*: Steingass, p. 1370; Wehr, p. 936. For this answer, cf. Ibn Wāfid, p. 21 (Arabic) and p. 59 (Spanish).

227 *Amīr bārīs*: *Tuḥfa*, p. 12; Dozy, I, 37.

228 *Bizr qaṭūnā*: al-Kindī, pp. 317–18.

granate flower,[229] gum tragacanth,[230] plantain,[231] horned poppy,[232] sumac,[233] boxthorn,[234] gallnut,[235] black nightshade,[236] gum arabic, *rāmik*,[237] and ribes.[238]

QUESTION NINETEEN: **[28b]** How many cold and moist medicines in the second degree does Ibn Wāfid mention?

ANSWER: Nine (*sic*). They are blite,[239] watermelon (*biṭṭīkh*),[240] cucumber (*qiththā'*),[241] henna, watermelon,[242] sea moss,[243] truffles,[244] apricots,[245] pumpkin,[246] lettuce,[247] and peaches.[248]

QUESTION TWENTY: How many useful, hot and dry medicines in the third degree are there? How many are hot and moist, cold and dry, and cold and moist?

ANSWER: As for hot and dry medicines in the third degree in Ibn Wāfid's book, their number is eighty-three (*sic*). They are asafetida,[249] anise,[250] feverfew,[251] wild ginger (*asārūn*),[252] savin,[253] dodder (*afthīmūn*),

---

229 *Jullinār*: *ibid*., pp. 253–54; al-Samarqandī, p. 185; *EI* ², *Supplement*, *s.v.* "Djullanār" (Dietrich).

230 *Kathīrā'*: al-Kindī, p. 323; al-Dīnawarī, *al-Nabāt*, II, 234; al-Samarqandī, p. 196.

231 *Lisān al-ḥamal*: Maimonides, no. 213; al-Samarqandī, p. 224; *Tuḥfa*, p. 108.

232 *Māmīthā*: al-Kindī, p. 332; al-Samarqandī, p. 224.

233 *Summāq*: al-Kindī, p. 285; al-Samarqandī, p. 178.

234 *'Awsaj*: al-Kindī, p. 308; Wehr, p. 657.

235 *'Afṣ*: al-Kindī, p. 305; al-Samarqandī, p. 238; *EI* ², *s.v.* "'Afṣ" (L. Kopf).

236 *'Inab al-tha'lab*: al-Kindī, p. 307; al-Samarqandī, p. 203.

237 Al-Kindī, pp. 270–71, calls it an electuary of gallnut with aromatic drugs; *Tuḥfa*, p. 157, "confection."

238 *Rībās*: al-Samarqandī, p. 177. For this answer, cf. Ibn Wāfid, p. 21 (Arabic) and p. 59 (Spanish).

239 *Baqla yamāniyya*: *Tuḥfa*, pp. 31–32; al-Samarqandī, p. 241.

240 Al-Samarqandī, p. 215.

241 *Ibid*., p. 219.

242 Hava, p. 214; Wehr, p. 290.

243 *Ṭuḥlub*: *Tuḥfa*, p. 90; Steingass, p. 810; Hava, p. 427; Levey, *Toxicology*, p. 123.

244 *Kam'a*: *Tuḥfa*, p. 99; Steingass, 1048; Hava, p. 664; Levey, *Toxicology*, p. 123.

245 *Mishmish*: al-Samarqandī, pp. 197–98; *EI* ², *s.v.* "Mishmish" (Viré).

246 *Qar'*: al-Kindī, pp. 314–15; al-Samarqandī, p. 189.

247 *Khass*: al-Samarqandī, pp. 29, 189.

248 For this answer, cf. Ibn Wāfid, p. 21 (Arabic) and p. 60 (Spanish).

249 *Anjudān*: *Tuḥfa*, pp. 10–11, 77; Steingass, pp. 106, 115.

250 *Anīsūn*: al-Kindī, p. 237; al-Samarqandī, p. 173.

251 *Aqḥuwān*: al-Samarqandī, p. 230.

252 Al-Kindī, p. 227; al-Samarqandī, p. 223.

253 *Abhul*: al-Samarqandī, p. 208.

potash,[254] polypody,[255] arthanita,[256] orchis (*būzaydān*),[257] elder, Arabian jasmine, Indian quince,[258] opoponax,[259] gentian,[260] pearl millet (*dukhān*),[261] wild carrot,[262] Chinese cinnamon,[263] hypericum,[264] gum ammoniac,[265] sweet flag,[266] *zarnab*,[267] pitch,[268] artichoke,[269] white chameleon,[270] black chameleon,[271] Greek walnut,[272] lousewort,[273] ben nut,[274] amomum,[275] juniper nut,[276] thyme,[277] colocynth,[278] scammony (*ḥabb al-nīl*),[279] danewort,[280] harmel,[281] peucedanum,[282] cumin,[283]

---

254 *Ushnān*: al-Kindī, pp. 231–32; al-Samarqandī, p. 237; Lane, *Lexicon*, I.1, 62.

255 *Basfānij*: al-Kindī, p. 243; al-Samarqandī, p. 201.

256 *Bakhūr maryam*: *Tuḥfa*, p. 41; Steingass, p. 160; Lane, *Lexicon*, I.1, 159.

257 Al-Samarqandī, pp. 190–91.

258 *Bull wa-full wa-shull*: Dozy, I, 107, II, 276, and I, 780 respectively. Cf. Steingass, p. 936 for *full* and p. 757 for *shull*. Maimonides, no. 57, gives *ball wa-shall* as spices of the elder tree.

259 *Jāwashīr*: al-Samarqandī, p. 207; Steingass, p. 354.

260 *Janṭiyānā*: al-Samarqandī, p. 192; *Tuḥfa*, p. 47.

261 Cf. n. 131 above.

262 *Dūqū*: al-Kindī, p. 269; al-Samarqandī, p. 199; *Tuḥfa*, pp. 52–53.

263 *Dār ṣīnī*: al-Kindī, pp. 265–66; al-Samarqandī, pp. 171, 194; *EI* ², *Supplement*, *s.v.* "Dār Ṣīnī" (Dietrich).

264 *Hiyūfārīqūn*: Maimonides, no. 115; *Tuḥfa*, pp. 57–58.

265 *Wushshāq*: *Tuḥfa*, p. 62; Dozy, II, 808; Steingass, p. 1469.

266 *Wajj*: al-Kindī, pp. 343–44; al-Samarqandī, pp. 27, 198–99, 222.

267 Various meanings, cf. al-Kindī, p. 274, yew; Hava, p. 288, Egyptian willow and others; Levey, *Toxicology*, p. 120, zedoary.

268 *Zift*: al-Kindī, p. 276.

269 *Ḥarshaf*: Dozy, I, 271; Steingass, p. 415.

270 *Ḥāmālāwun lawqus*: Gunther, *Dioscorides*, p. 243; Dubler, *Materia Médica*, II, 243.

271 *Ḥāmālāwun mālas*: Gunther, *Dioscorides*, 243; Dubler, *Materia Médica*, II, 243–44.

272 *Jawz rūmī*: Steingass, p. 377.

273 *Ḥabb al-ra's*: *Tuḥfa*, p. 115; Dozy, I, 240.

274 *Ḥabb al-bān*: al-Kindī, p. 241; al-Samarqandī, p. 243. Cf. Kazimirski, I, 363.

275 *Ḥamāmā*: *Tuḥfa*, p. 75; Steingass, p. 430; Levey, *Toxicology*, p. 118.

276 *Ḥabb ʿarʿar*: Dozy, I, 240; Steingass, p. 844; Hava, p. 461.

277 *Ḥāshā'*: al-Kindī, p. 256; al-Samarqandī, p. 29.

278 *Ḥanẓal*: al-Kindī, p. 262; al-Samarqandī, p. 196.

279 Dozy, I, 241; Kazimirski, I, 364; Hava, p. 108. Cf. Steingass, p. 410.

280 *Khāmā aqṭī*: Steingass, p. 442.

281 *Ḥarmal*: al-Kindī, p. 258; al-Samarqandī, p. 206.

282 *Yarbaṭūra*: Maimonides, no. 33; *Tuḥfa*, pp. 94–95, *yarbaṭūn*.

283 *Kammūn*: al-Kindī, pp. 327–28; al-Samarqandī, p. 191; *EI* ², *s.v.* "Kammūn" (G.S. Colin).

cubeb,[284] caraway,[285] celery,[286] —,[287] pissasphalt, Jewish bdellium,[288] hoarhound,[289] bean trefoil,[290] marjoram,[291] royal cumin,[292] mint (*na'na'*),[293] serpolet,[294] rue,[295] **[29a]** cinnamon,[296] sagapenum,[297] scammony (*saqmūniyyā*),[298] squill,[299] *'akūb*,[300] *'urūq*,[301] radish,[302] —,[303] hart's tongue,[304] chaste tree, mint (*fawtanaj*),[305] colophony,[306] wild thyme, great centaury,[307] small centaury,[308] bastard cardamom,[309] southernwood,[310] costus,[311] clove,[312] galbanum,[313] cochineal,[314]

---

284 *Kabbāba*: al-Kindī, pp. 321–22; al-Samarqandī, p. 193.

285 *Karāwiyā*: al-Samarqandī, p. 199; Steingass, p. 1020; Hava, p. 653.

286 *Karafs*: al-Kindī, pp. 324–25; al-Samarqandī, pp. 173, 200.

287 Word unidentified, see Arabic text.

288 *Muql al-yahūd*: Levey, *Toxicology*, p. 126. See n. 143 above.

289 *Marrūya*: Hava, p. 717.

290 *Yanbūt*: al-Kindī, p. 345; al-Dīnawarī, *al-Nabāt*, II, 349–51; al-Samarqandī, p. 196.

291 *Marzanjūsh*: al-Kindī, p. 353.

292 *Nānakhwāt*: *ibid.*, p. 339; al-Samarqandī, p. 185.

293 Maimonides, no. 256; Steingass, p. 1412.

294 *Nammām*: al-Samarqandī, p. 209; Steingass, p. 1425; Hava, p. 800.

295 *Sadhāb*: *Tuhfa*, p. 159; Steingass, p. 664; Hava, p. 315; Levey, *Toxicology*, p. 120.

296 *Salīkha*: al-Samarqandī, p. 194.

297 *Sakabīnaj*: *ibid.*, p. 207.

298 *Ibid.*, p. 196.

299 *'Unṣul*: *ibid.*, pp. 172, 219.

300 Various meanings: cf. Dozy, II, 155, *'akkūb*; Steingass, p. 861.

301 "Roots," various kinds: cf. al-Kindī, p. 303; Dozy, II, 119; Steingass, p. 846; Lane, *Lexicon*, I.5, 2018–19.

302 *Fujl*: Dozy, II, 243; Levey, *Toxicology*, p. 123.

303 Word unidentified, see Arabic text.

304 *Isqilīnūs*: Steingass, p. 58, *isqilīnus*.

305 Al-Kindī, pp. 312–13; al-Samarqandī, p. 201.

306 *Qulfūniyya*: al-Kindī, p. 318; Maimonides, no. 352, *qulfūniyā*.

307 *Qanṭūriyūn kabīr*: al-Kindī, p. 319; al-Samarqandī, p. 201.

308 *Qanṭūriyūn daqīq*.

309 *Qardamānā*: al-Samarqandī, pp. 199, 229.

310 *Qayṣūm*: *ibid.*, p. 205.

311 *Quṣṭ*: al-Kindī, p. 316, and al-Samarqandī, p. 199, both spell it *qusṭ*. Cf. Levey, *Toxicology*, p. 124.

312 *Qaranful*: al-Kindī, pp. 215–16; al-Samarqandī, pp. 179–80; *EI*², *s.v.* "Ḳaranful" (E. Ashtor).

313 *Qinna*: al-Kindī, p. 319; al-Samarqandī, pp. 235–36.

314 *Qirmiz*: Steingass, p. 966.

betonica,[315] cardamine,[316] fennel,[317] dill,[318] sowbread,[319] black cumin,[320] wormwood (*shīḥ*),[321] turpeth,[322] garlic,[323] galingale,[324] the two hellebores,[325] sweet bay,[326] leopard's bane,[327] hyssop, and pine resin.[328] As for hot and moist medicines in the third degree, there are four. They are ginger,[329] root of the rush-nut,[330] elecampane,[331] and thapsia.[332] As for cold and dry medicines in the third degree, there are nine. They are henbane,[333] dragon's blood plant,[334] mandrake,[335] camphor,[336] areca nut,[337] sandalwood,[338] hemlock,[339] tamarind,[340] and tabasheer.[341] As for cold and moist medicines in the third degree, there are four. They are common purslane,[342] sempervivum,[343] knotweed,[344] and toadstool.[345]

---

315 *Qasiṭran*: *Tuḥfa*, pp. 41–42.
316 *Qurrat al-ʿayn*: *ibid.*, p. 147; Dozy, II, 319; Hava, p. 595.
317 *Rāziyanaj*: al-Samarqandī, p. 173.
318 *Shabath*: al-Kindī, p. 292; al-Samarqandī, p. 231; *EI* 2, *s.v.* "Shibithth" (Dietrich).
319 *Shajarat maryam*: *Tuḥfa*, pp. 29, 104–105; Dozy, I, 730; Steingass, p. 735.
320 *Shūnīz*: al-Samarqandī, p. 240.
321 Al-Kindī, p. 296; al-Samarqandī, p. 182.
322 *Turbad*: al-Kindī, p. 52; al-Samarqandī, p. 171.
323 *Thūm*: al-Kindī, p. 251; al-Samarqandī, p. 242.
324 *Khūlanjān*: al-Samarqandī, p. 182.
325 *Kharbaqān*, black and white: Maimonides, no. 399; Steingass, p. 452.
326 *Ghār*: al-Kindī, pp. 308–309; al-Samarqandī, p. 192.
327 *Durūnj*: al-Kindī, p. 267.
328 *Rātinaj*: *ibid.*, p. 269; al-Samarqandī, p. 235.
329 *Zanjabīl*: al-Kindī, p. 277; al-Samarqandī, pp. 29, 186.
330 *Ḥabb al-zalam*: *Tuḥfa*, pp. 84–85; Dozy, I, 240. Cf. Steingass, p. 620.
331 *Rāsin*: al-Kindī, p. 270; al-Samarqandī, p. 229.
332 *Tāfsiyā*: al-Samarqandī, p. 240; Levey, *Toxicology*, p. 117.
333 *Banj*: al-Kindī, p. 246; *EI* 2, *s.v.* "Bandj" (Meyerhof).
334 *Dam al-akhawayn*: al-Kindī, p. 268; al-Samarqandī, pp. 213–14.
335 *Yabrūḥ*: Gunther, *Dioscorides*, p. 473; Dubler, *Materia Médica*, II, 338–40; al-Samarqandī, pp. 186, 234; *EI* 2, *s.v.* "Yabrūḥ" (Penelope C. Johnstone).
336 *Kāfūr*: al-Kindī, p. 321; al-Samarqandī, p. 171; *EI* 2, *s.v.* "Kāfūr" (Dietrich).
337 *Fawfal*: al-Kindī, p. 313; al-Samarqandī, pp. 223–24.
338 *Ṣandal*: al-Kindī, p. 298; al-Samarqandī, p. 183; *EI* 2, *s.v.* "Ṣandal" (Dietrich).
339 *Shawkarān*: al-Kindī, pp. 295–96.
340 *Tamar hindī*: *ibid.*, p. 251; al-Samarqandī, pp. 183–84.
341 *Ṭabāshīr*: al-Kindī, p. 300; al-Samarqandī, p. 179; *EI* 2, *s.v.* "Ṭabāshīr" (Dietrich).
342 *Baqlat ḥamqāʾ*: al-Kindī, pp. 244–45.
343 *Ḥayy al-ʿālam*: al-Samarqandī, p. 241.
344 *ʿAṣā l-rāʿī*: *ibid.*, pp. 230–31.
345 *Fuṭr*: *Tuḥfa*, p. 141; Hava, p. 568; Levey, *Toxicology*, p. 123. For this answer, cf. Ibn Wāfid, p. 22 (Arabic) and pp. 61–66 (Spanish).

CHAPTER SIX

ON TREATMENT, COMPRISING TWENTY QUESTIONS

QUESTION ONE: How many [kinds of] symptoms are meant to be treated and what is it that indicates what they will be?

ANSWER: This is recorded in the fifty-ninth book **[29b]** of al-Masīḥī's *al-Kutub al-Mi'a*,[1] where he says: They are five. The first is the symptom that reveals the nature of what is to be used for treatment, and the kind of illness indicates what it will be. The second is the symptom that reveals the amount of what is to be used for treatment. What indicates this is the temperament of the body, the scope of the illness, and the status of everything that provides therapeutic guidance one way or another. The third is the symptom that reveals the time during which treatment is to be carried out. What indicates this is how long the illness lasts, how strong it is, and the condition of everything that provides therapeutic guidance one way or another. The fourth is the symptom that reveals how this method of treatment is to be used. The fifth is the symptom that reveals the selection of the substance that is to be used for treatment. What indicates these last two symptoms are the illness, temperament, [vital] faculty, and everything that provides therapeutic guidance one way or another, namely, location, time of day, and weather conditions.

QUESTION TWO: How many procedures are there for treating the symptoms of each one of the organs in particular and how is each treatment done?

ANSWER: This is recorded in the fifty-ninth book of al-Masīḥī's *al-Kutub al-Mi'a*. Four. The first is the method understood from the condition of the ailing organ. The second is the method understood from its physiognomy. The third is the method understood **[30a]** from its position. And the fourth is the method understood from its strength. As for the method understood from the condition of the ailing organ, examples are all the organs in which heat is predominant, like the flesh, or in which coldness is predominant, like the nerves, or which are in between, like the skin.

---

[1] On Abū Sahl 'Īsā ibn Yaḥyā al-Masīḥī (d. 401/1010) and his *al-Kutub al-mi'a fī l-ṣināʿa al-ṭibbiyya* ["The One Hundred Books on the Medical Art"], see *GAL* I, 238 and *S* I, 423–24; *GAS* III, 326–27; Ullmann, *Medizin*, p. 151. According to *GAS*, this work was published in Hyderabad in 1959 under a different title and author. We have not seen this book.

If the natural temperament of any one of them changes, it needs to be returned to what it was by things that incline away from balance in the opposite direction to which it has inclined. As for the method understood from the physiognomy of the organ, some organs are hollow like the stomach, and some are not; some are solid, like the nerves of the hands and feet, and some are hollow internally and externally together, like the lungs, which are surrounded by the chest on the exterior and on the interior by the windpipe and pulsating veins (arteries) scattering from it. When the organ is deep and porous like the lungs, it cannot bear being treated with strong medications. When it is compact and firm like the two kidneys, it can bear strong medications. When it is medium like the liver, the medication must be moderate. As for the procedure with regard to the position of the organ, it is to look at the location of the organ in treating its poor condition because, if it is near, the medication can reach it and the strength of the medication will remain unchanged. If it is distant, the medication cannot reach it without passing through other organs, so one must increase the strength of the medicine by the amount it will lose **[30b]** on the way to the organ. As for the procedure with regard to the strength of the organ, it is to determine if it works generally to the benefit of the entire body, like the stomach or diaphragm, and to determine if it is responsive to sensation in the way that the eye is. When it is necessary for us to treat the liver or stomach with a dressing that penetrates, we mix the penetrating medications with an adhesive and fragrant medication, so that the strength of the medication remains the same.

QUESTION THREE: How many steps are [followed] in treatment with medications?

ANSWER: This is recorded in the *Kulliyyāt al-Qānūn*. Three. The first is the rule of choosing its quality, that is, choosing it with regard to hotness, coldness, wetness, or dryness. The second is the rule of choosing its amount (dose), which is divided into the rule of estimating its weight and the rule of estimating its quality (i.e., degree of hotness, etc.). The third is the rule of determining its time [of administration].[2]

QUESTION FOUR: How many conditions do you consider with regard to drawing out [the substance of the illness]?

ANSWER: This is recorded in the *Kulliyyāt al-Qānūn*. Four. The first is [to consider] the opposite direction, such as drawing out from right to left

[2] *Al-Qānūn*, I, 188. Cf. Gruner, *Canon*, p. 463; Shah, *Principles*, p. 361.

(i.e., if the substance is going to the right, it should be drawn out from the left) and from top to bottom. The second is to consider what [part of the body] is associated [physiologically] with it. Thus, menstruation is suppressed by placing cupping glasses on the breasts in order to draw out what is associated with it. The third is to consider what is parallel to it. Thus, one bleeds the right basilic vein for an illness of the liver, and bleeds the left basilic vein for an illness of the spleen. The fourth is to consider the distance, so that **[31a]** the attractee (i.e., the member into which morbid substances are drawn) will not be closer than the attractor (i.e., the diseased member).[3]

QUESTION FIVE: How many essential considerations are there in preparing medications and what are some examples?

ANSWER: This is recorded in al-Rāzī's *al-Fuṣūl*.[4] Five. First, sometimes a medication that is of benefit against a certain illness and strengthens a certain organ can harm another [organ]. Thus, one has to prepare something with it that will prevent this. An example of this is when we mix castoreum with opium, so that it does not become highly injurious. Second, if a medication does not go to the place we desire, we have to mix it with something that will take it there. An example is when we mix fine aromas with medicinal clay[5] and gum arabic for someone who coughs blood from the lungs and chest. Third, if a medication is useful against a certain illness but part of it is more useful to some bodies and temperaments than others, and the doctor is primarily interested in a medication that will remedy that illness, and the doctor wants to have a medication that would be good to use for many illnesses, then he must prepare that medication from medications useful against a variety of illnesses, like the theriac[6] that is useful for many kinds of sicknesses. Fourth, sometimes it is necessary to expell different humors from the body. Thus, one must prepare a medication for this from medications each of which expells one of the humors. An example is Galen's pills known as *al-qūqāyā*

---

[3] *Al-Qānūn*, I, 189. Cf. Gruner, *Canon*, p. 466; Shah, *Principles*, p. 363; Ḥunayn, pp. 5, 94.

[4] On Abū Bakr Muḥammad ibn Zakariyyā' al-Rāzī (d. 311/923), known as Rhazes in the West, and his *Kitāb al-Murshid aw al-Fuṣūl* ["The Guide, or Aphorisms"], see *GAL* I, 233–35, and *S* I, 417–21; *GAS* III, 274–78, 284; Ullmann, *Medizin*, pp. 128–30, index; *EI*², *s.v.* "al-Rāzī" (P. Kraus and S. Pines); Dodge, *Fihrist*, II, 701–709. *Al-Murshid* was edited by Albert Z. Iskandar in *Majallat Ma'had al-Makhṭūṭāt al-'Arabiyya* 7 (1961), 1–125.

[5] *Ṭīn makhtūm*: literally "stamped clay," presumably meaning that it was the genuine product. There were different kinds, see *Tuḥfa*, p. 88.

[6] On theriac, see Leiser and Dols, "Evliyā Chelebi's Description of Medicine," pt. 1, pp. 209–15.

prepared from aloe (*ṣabir*), scammony (*saqmūniyā*), **[31b]** colocynth pulp, and extract of wormwood (*afsintīn*). Fifth, sometimes a useful medication is not used unless it is dissolved in something else, like litharge and all hard medications which cannot be used in ointments until they are dissolved in [edible] oil and *khulūl*.[7] They are prepared and melted with gum arabic and fat.[8]

QUESTION SIX: How many kinds of treatment are there for bad temperament (dyscrasia, a bad mixture of the humors)?

ANSWER: This is recorded in the *Kulliyyāt al-Qānūn*. Three. First, if the bad temperament is deep-rooted (chronic), its treatment is with an absolutely opposite acting [drug]. This is the absolute treatment. Second, if it occurs at the termination of the event (illness), its remedy and treatment are by preservation [of the health by taking the necessary measures] in advance and this prevents the cause. Third, if it is about to occur, one need only prevent the cause, and it is (also ?) called preservation in advance.[9]

QUESTION SEVEN: How many things should be properly considered with regard to evacuation?

ANSWER: This is recorded in the *Kulliyyāt al-Qānūn*. Ten (*sic*). They are plethora, [vital] faculty, temperament, indicative symptoms, appearance, age, season, climate and country, [patient's] habit of evacuation, and occupation.[10]

QUESTION EIGHT: How many things should be considered with regard to any case of induced evacuation?

ANSWER: This is recorded in the *Kulliyyāt al-Qānūn*. Five. First, to evacuate [only] what [substance] should be evacuated, which must be followed **[32a]** by rest. Second, one should consider the direction of its predilection. For example, nausea is treated by vomiting, and colic by purgation. Third, [one should consider] the direction of predilection of the emitting organ. For example, [one has to consider] the right basilic and not the right cephalic for illnesses of the liver. If one makes a mistake in this, it can cause harm. Moreover, the emitting organ must be baser [than that which is to be evacuated], so that the [morbid] substance will not have

---

[7] *Khall* is vinegar, but *duhn khall* is sesame seed oil: *Tuḥfa*, p. 56. The last two words in this sentence are *bi-l-adhān wa-l-khulūl*, i.e., the plurals of *duhn* and *khall*.

[8] Al-Rāzī, *al-Murshid*, pp. 61–62.

[9] *Al-Qānūn*, I, 191. Cf. Gruner, *Canon*, p. 470; Shah, *Principles*, p. 366.

[10] *Al-Qānūn*, I, 192. Cf. Gruner, *Canon*, p. 472; Shah, *Principles*, pp. 368–69.

a predilection for what is nobler. Its emission from it must be natural, like the urinary organs, thanks to the convexity of the liver, and the intestines, thanks to their concavity. Sometimes the organ from which it (the morbid substance) emerges is the organ that needs to be evacuated. But it may have a disease so that it is necessary to go to another. Fourth, the time of evacuation. Galen insisted that chronic illnesses must be left to ripen before evacuation, and afterwards it is necessary to drink sedatives. As for acute illnesses, it is also best to wait for ripening, especially if they (the humors) are quiescent. If they are active, promptly evacuating the [morbid] substance [of the humors] is preferable because the harm from their activity is greater than the harm from evacuating them prior to the time that they ripen. This is especially so if the humors are thin or if it (the morbid substance of the humor) is in the hollows of the veins and does not enter the organs. If the humor is confined within an organ, it will not move at all until it ripens and has a moderate status.[11]

QUESTION NINE: If several illnesses occur together, with which treatments should you begin?

ANSWER: This is recorded in *al-Kulliyyāt*. You begin with what pertains to one of three characteristics. **[32b]** First, with the one which, if not itself cured, the second will not be cured, like an inflamation and an ulcer. If these two occur together, we would treat the inflamation first until the [bad] temperament accompanying it disappears. But the ulcer would not be healed, so then the ulcer is treated. Second, if one is the cause of the other, such as an obstruction and a fever, we would treat the obstruction first and then the fever. We cannot influence the fever because it is not possible for the fever to disappear while its cause is there. Its treatment is to dry it, which attacks the fever. Third, if one of the two is more serious, such as if synochus combines with hemiplegia, we would treat the synochus by extinguishing [the heat] and bleeding and not pay attention to the hemiplegia. If the illness and symptoms are combined, we start treating the illness unless the symptom predominates. Then, we go straight to that symptom and we ignore the illness as when we give narcotics for extremely painful colic, if it becomes difficult, and even if it aggravates the colic itself.[12]

QUESTION TEN: How many uses are there for oxymel?

---

[11] *Al-Qānūn*, I, 192–93. Cf. Gruner, *Canon*, pp. 473–75; Shah, *Principles*, pp. 369–70.

[12] *Al-Qānūn*, I, 221. Cf. Gruner, *Canon*, pp. 529–30; Shah, *Principles*, pp. 422–23.

ANSWER: This is recorded in Ibn al-Mudawwar's *al-Tajārib*[13] cited from Ḥunayn's treatise *Fī l-Sakanjubīn*.[14] Eighty-eight uses. First, it cools a temperament inclining toward excessive heat and moderates it by extinguishing and calming that heat. Second, if it is drunk pure, it protects a cold body. Third, if it is drunk in a copious mixture of which it is one-fourth and water is three-fourths, it will make a dry body moist. Fourth, it dries a moist body by cutting the moisture **[33a]** and reducing it in the body; it expels it if it is drunk pure, and especially if it is heated. Fifth, it is useful against periodic tertian fever. Sixth, it is useful against continuous tertian fever. Seventh, it is useful against paroxysmal quartan fever. Eighth, it is useful against hectic fever. Ninth, it is useful against continuous quotidian fever. Tenth, it is useful against paroxysmal quotidian fever. Eleventh, it is useful against the remittent fever known as synochus, which is bloody. Twelfth, it is useful against ardent fever. Thirteenth, it is useful against the fever composed of phlegmatic fever and continuous tertian fever. Fourteenth, it is useful against the fever composed of continuous phlegmatic fever and paroxysmal phlegmatic fever. Fifteenth, it is useful against the fever composed of continuous tertian fever and paroxysmal tertian fever. Sixteenth, it is useful against the fever composed of continuous phlegmatic fever and paroxysmal tertian fever, which is semi-tertian fever. Eighteenth,[15] it is useful against a combination of paroxysmal tertian fever and quartan fever. Nineteenth, it is useful against a combination of paroxysmal quartan fever and continuous quartan fever. Twentieth, it is useful against a combination of continuous tertian fever and continuous quartan fever. Twenty-first, it is useful against a combination of continuous tertian fever and paroxysmal quartan fever. Twenty-second, it is useful against a combination of paroxysmal tertian fever and continuous quartan fever. Twenty-third, it is useful against a combination of intermittent paroxysmal tertian fever and intermittent phlegmtic fever and intermittant quartan fever. Twenty-fourth, it is useful against **[33b]** a combination of intermittent phlegmatic fever and intermittent tertian fever. Twenty-fifth, it is useful against a com-

[13] The identification of this author and his work ["Experiences," probably in the sense of case notes], is not certain. See Dietrich, *Medicinalia*, p. 198 n. 1; Ullmann, *Medizin*, p. 310.

[14] On Ḥunayn ibn Isḥāq (d. 260/873), see *GAL* I, 205–206, and *S* I, 366–69; *GAS* III, 247–56; Ullmann, *Medizin*, pp. 115–19, index; *EI*², *s.v.* "Ḥunayn b. Isḥāḳ al-ʿIbādī" (G. Strohmaier); Dodge, *Fihrist*, II, 693–94. We have no record of a book by him entitled *Fī l-Sakanjubīn* ["On Oxymel"], but it may well be lost or part of another of his numerous works.

[15] The seventeenth is missing.

bination of continuous phlegmatic fever and intermittent quartan fever. Twenty-eighth,[16] it is useful against all kinds of putrid fevers of the humors, which it dissolves and removes. Twenty-ninth, it is useful against hectic fever that occurs in the moisture in the internal organs. Thirtieth, it is useful against hectic fever that occurs in moist organs. Thirty-first, it is useful against hectic fever that occurs in the moisture found within the basic organs themselves. Thirty-second, it is useful against ephemeral fever resulting from fatigue. Thirty-third, it is useful against ephemeral fever resulting from intoxication. Thirty-fourth, it is useful against ephemeral fever resulting from indigestion. Thirty-fifth, it is useful against ephemeral fever resulting from extreme coldness. Thirty-sixth, it is useful against ephemeral fever resulting from the burning sun and the summer's extremely hot wind. Thirty-seventh, it is useful against ephemeral fever resulting from the thickening of the surface of the body, as happens to someone whose skin has been reddened by alum. Thirty-eighth, it is useful against fever resulting from insomnia caused by grief. Thirty-ninth, it is useful against ephemeral fever resulting from anxiety and sorrow. Fortieth, it is useful against ephemeral fever resulting from sleeplessness the cause of which is unknown. Forty-first, it is useful against ephemeral fever resulting from a lover **[34a]** or from painful words or separation [from a loved one]. Forty-second, it is useful against all other mixed fevers. Forty-third, it is useful against fainting resulting from plethora, which blocks the layers. Forty-fourth, it is useful against fainting resulting from bad temperament. Forty-fifth, it is useful against fainting resulting from pain. Forty-sixth, it is useful against constriction of the uterus. Forty-seventh, it is useful against stroke and swooning if one gargles with it in pure form and rubs the throat with it and *iyārij fiqarā*.[17] Forty-eighth, it is useful against the burning sensation in the stomach. Forty-ninth, it is useful against fainting occurring at the beginning of an attack of fever. Fiftieth, it is useful against cerebral disease. Fifty-first, it is useful against pleurisy (*birsām*). Fifty-second, it is useful against pleurisy (*dhāt al-janb*). Fifty-third, it is useful against pneumonia. Fifty-fourth, it is useful against a headache resulting from the sun. Fifty-fifth, it is useful against a headache resulting from gas caused by bad temperament that is hot and mixed with a substance [of an illness]. Fifty-sixth, it is useful against a headache resulting from a bad temperament that is cold and mixed with a substance [of an illness]. Fifty-seventh, it is useful against a headache resulting from a cold

16 The twenty-sixth and twenty-seventh are missing.

17 A compound electuary: al-Kindī, p. 238; al-Samarqandī, pp. 153, 196, 201.

wind. Fifty-eighth, it is useful against a headache **[34b]** resulting from drinking wine and hangover. Fifty-ninth, it is useful against bewilderment and dizziness. Sixtieth, it is useful against a headache following a pain in the cardia. Sixty-first, it is useful against long-lasting chronic migraines. Sixty-second, it is useful against phrenitis (*qarāniṭūs*). Sixty-third, it is useful against the pain in the brain caused by a burning hot humor and melancholia. Sixty-fourth, it is useful against trembling if taken pure. Sixty-fifth, it is useful against a cough caused by humidity if taken pure. Sixty-sixth, it is useful against obstructions in the veins between the liver and the gall bladder. Sixty-seventh, it opens the channels between the liver and the gall bladder. Sixty-eighth, it opens the channels between the liver and the spleen. Sixty-ninth, it opens the channels between the stomach and the gall bladder. Seventieth, it is useful against some forms of dropsy especially anasarca. Seventy-first, it disintegrates kidney stones if it is drunk pure with scorpion ashes (*ramād al-ʿaqārib?*). Seventy-second, it is useful against chancres. Seventy-third, it is useful against boils on the body. Seventy-fourth, it is useful against pimples and ulcers, especially at the joints. Seventy-fifth, it is useful against pain **[35a]** in the joints caused by hot substances. Seventy-sixth, it dislodges and restricts sticky phlegm, which coats the entire stomach, and makes it descend. Seventy-seventh, it eliminates the yellow bile when it accumulates in the stomach and remains for a long time. Seventy-eighth, it is useful against acutely itching (prurigo) mange. Seventy-ninth, it is of wondrous use against excitability and calms it. Eightieth, it opens the obstructions occurring in the channels of the spleen. Eighty-first, it is useful against inflamations of the liver. Eighty-second, it is useful for palpitation occurring in the heart. Eighty-third, it makes the black bile, which is congested in the stomach, descend. Eighty-fourth, it is useful against smallpox and measles. Eighty-fifth, it is useful against ulcers of the bladder. Eighty-sixth, it is useful against poor respiration and poor tumescence. Eighty-seventh, it makes the menstrual discharge (menses) descend if a numbness occurs when it takes place. Eighty-eighth, it helps keep the uterus from going to one side.

QUESTION ELEVEN: How much do people praise slightly acidic oxymel?

ANSWER: This is recorded in the *Masāʾil al-Najjād*,[18] where the author says: If it is used, the mouth and palate become moist to make the acidity

[18] This work ["The Problems Posed by al-Najjād"] is unidentified; see Dietrich, *Medicinalia*, p. 198. Perhaps the same work as indicated in Chapter 10 n. 10 below.

in the yellow bile abate. It helps to spit phlegm **[35b]** and abate the thirst, is beneficial to everything in the hypochondrium, and prevents the occurrence of intestinal harm because the nature of the intestines is cold, dry, and sinewy.

QUESTION TWELVE: For what reason is [a patient] ordered to drink oxymel during acute illnesses two hours before drinking barley water and two hours afterwards?

ANSWER: This is recorded in the *Masā'il al-Najjād*. As for before-hand, it removes and extinguishes the flame. As for afterwards, it consumes what the barley water generates.

QUESTION THIRTEEN: What is the general principle regarding treatment of putrid fever?

ANSWER: This is recorded in Ibn Sīnā's *al-Juz'iyyāt*, where he says: The aim in treating these fevers is sometimes directed toward the fever, in which case it needs to be cold and moist, and sometimes it is directed toward the substance [of the illness], in which case it needs to ripen or be purged. Ripening of what is thick can be corrected by thinning, and ripening of what is thin can be corrected by thickening. Sometimes the cooling of the fever and the ripening of the humor are in opposition. In this case, it is necessary to keep an eye on the more important of the two. If the [vital] faculty is good, you eliminate the cause, cool the humor, and cut off nourishment. If it is poor, you work on adjusting the opposite. Then you make it cold and revive the [vital] faculty by nourishment.[19]

QUESTION FOURTEEN: What is the general principle for the treatment of the five sicknesses of the nerves, that is, numbness, **[36a]** spasms, tremors, quivering, and hemiplegia?

ANSWER: This is recorded in the *Juz'iyyāt al-Qānūn* of Ibn Sīnā, who indicates that one should bleed [the patient] at the back of the brain and not hasten to use strong medications. Rather, one should restrict oneself to gentle things that soften and ripen. Enemas are also good. Afterwards, one uses strong purgatives. From the beginning, the hemiplegic should be fed honey water or barley water for two or three days and, if the strength holds up, until the fourteenth day and then try to starve him and make him thirsty.[20]

---

19 *Al-Qānūn*, III, 21.
20 *Ibid.*, II, 93.

QUESTION FIFTEEN: What is the difference between medication and nourishment?

ANSWER: This is recorded in Ibn Riḍwān's *al-Uṣūl*, where he says: The difference between nourishment and medication is that nourishment changes in the body. Its chyle changes until it becomes one of the gastric juices in the body. Some nourishments change quickly like wine, some change at a medium rate like bread, and some change slowly like beef. Some change the body at first and then return, but then are changed by the body. Their chyle changes into some of the gastric juices of the body. An example is lettuce. Whatever behaves like this is called medicinal nourishment. Medication is whatever changes the body. Some changes the body and then returns and is changed by the body and is returned to it. This is called nutritional medication, like a sweet medicine. Some changes the body and then its strength decreases little by little; either the nature of the body rejects it **[36b]** and expels the medication from the body, or the medication is divided, changed, and its strength eliminated. This is called unrestricted medication. Some changes the body but does not differ from the body. This is called aggressive medication.

QUESTION SIXTEEN: What is the general principle for treating vomiting?

ANSWER: This is recorded in Ibn Sīnā's *al-Juz'iyyāt*, where he says: If vomiting is caused by the spoiling of used food, then improve the diet and assist it with hot fragrant strengtheners of the stomach. If its cause is a bad substance or an abundance of substance, that substance is expelled according to the principles of purging. Enemas are good for this. Vomiting will also stop vomiting if it is the result of a thick substance. Then, we make it gentle. Then, we stop it and purge it. Attracting the aggravating substance to the extremities is very useful in controlling the vomiting. If the nature is dry, the vomiting should only be controlled with a small amount of dry costives without injury. If the patient expells a strong medication that controls vomiting, repeat it once more. If he strongly dislikes it, change its odor or color. If nausea results while on an empty stomach, then the patient should have a full stomach and then be made to vomit. Most nausea caused by heat and dryness disappears by using dressings that cool and moisten. As for material (i.e., on a full stomach) nausea, it is necessary to purify it with something appropriate. The remaining problem should be treated with an antidote like fragrant medicines with hot and cold robs according to the type.[21]

[21] *Ibid.*, II, 339–40.

QUESTION SEVENTEEN: What is the difference between a dressing **[37a]** and a compress?

ANSWER: This is recorded in Ibn Riḍwān's *al-Uṣūl*. A compress is something hot applied [to an affected area] and a dressing is something cold applied [to affected area]. The purpose of both is to allow the [afflicted] organ to gain strength or make a change of humor until it returns to normal, or dissolve what has collected in it and ripen it, or push it backwards, or block what seeps out of, or flows out of, or heats parts of, the organ, or contract it, or soften it, or harden it, or make gentle, thicken, cut, or make sticky what occurs in it. The form of medication depends on which of these alternatives is desired.

QUESTION EIGHTEEN: How many characteristics are sought with regard to the use of medications that burn what burns and cleans what cleanses?

ANSWER: This is recorded among the words of Amīn al-Dawla Ibn al-Tilmīdh, who says: As for the characteristics that are sought with regard to what burns, there are five: either use something so that its sharpness is diminished, like yellow vitriol[22] or vitriol;[23] or something to acquire the sharpness, like quicklime;[24] or something to diminish its intensity, like crayfish (crab) and stag's horn;[25] or something to prepare it for being crushed, like silk;[26] or something to neutralize its bad essence. As for cleaning what cleanses, the characteristics that are sought for this are three: something to eliminate an acquired fiery feeling, like quicklime; something to make possible the washing out, like tutty;[27] and something to eliminate the intended strength, like the strength of making one faint resulting from the Armenian stone.[28]

QUESTION NINETEEN: What are the things that are harmful to the stomach and intestines?

ANSWER: This is recorded **[37b]** in the *Juz'iyyāt al-Qānūn*. Indigestion and plethora (overeating). Thus, the body of the glutton does not benefit because his food is not digested and the body does not benefit. The

---

22 *Qalqaṭār*: al-Kindī, p. 318; al-Samarqandī, p. 235.

23 *Zāj*: al-Kindī, p. 272; al-Samarqandī, p. 243.

24 *Nūra*: al-Kindī, p. 340; al-Samarqandī, p. 236.

25 *Qarn al-ayyil*: al-Kindī, p. 315; Wehr, p. 35.

26 *Ibrīsam*: *Tuḥfa*, p. 21.

27 *Tūtiyā*: al-Kindī, p. 250; al-Samarqandī, p. 224.

28 *Ḥajar armanī*: Steingass, p. 412. The answer to Question Eighteen probably comes from the *al-Aqrābādhīn* ["Materia Medica"] of Ibn al-Tilmīdh, see above Chapter 1 n. 9.

retention of gas and sediment is very injurious. Sometimes the sediment accumulates layer upon layer until it backs up to the stomach and causes great harm. All the juices that are not costive are especially bad. All [edible] oil loosens the stomach and is not suitable for it. The least harmful are olive oil and pistachio oil. Among the medications and food most harmful to the stomach are pine nuts, beets, grand basil, turnips without being boiled to shreds, sorrel, orache,[29] blite except with vinegar, garum, olive oil, fennugreek, and sesame. The latter two weaken the stomach. Milk[30] is harmful to the stomach and so are brains (*mikhākh* and *admigha*). With regard to drinks, whatever is viscous [is harmful]. And with regard to medication, juniper seeds, chast tree seeds,[31] and laxatives [are harmful]. Anything that is disliked is bad for the stomach. Coitus is among the most harmful things for the stomach. Violent vomiting, although it is beneficial from the point of view of purifying, is very harmful because it weakens the stomach.[32]

QUESTION TWENTY: What things are harmful to the liver?
ANSWER: This is recorded in Ibn Sīnā's *al-Juz'iyyāt*, where he says: Eating between meals and poor diet are among the most harmful things for the liver. Drinking cold water in one gulp on an empty stomach, after a bath, coitus, or exercise **[38a]** [is harmful] because it sometimes leads to an extreme cooling [of the liver] and this encourages an inflamed liver to contract quickly and substantially. Sometimes drinking a lot of cold water in this way leads to dropsy, in which case it should be mixed and not made very cold and should not be gulped but sipped little by little. All sticky things are harmful to the liver because they will cause an obstruction. Sweet drinks will cause an obstruction in the liver, although they clear what is in the chest.[33]

---

29 *Sarmaq*: al-Samarqandī, p. 216.
30 *Laban*: al-Kindī, p. 330.
31 *Ḥabb al-faqad*: al-Samarqandī, p. 175; Hava, p. 108.
32 *Al-Qānūn*, II, 306–307.
33 *Ibid.*, II, 355.

CHAPTER SEVEN

ON WHAT OPHTHALMOLOGISTS SHOULD BE ASKED, COMPRISING TWENTY QUESTIONS

QUESTION ONE: Licorice root should be used to anoint which eye diseases?

ANSWER: This is recorded from the words of Dioscorides as cited by Ibn Wāfid in his *al-Adwiya al-mufrada*, where he says: If the licorice root is peeled, pulverized, filtered with a fine sieve, and used as an ointment, it is useful medication for pterygium. It should be sprinkled on it. Then it consumes it, eliminates it, and eradicates all traces of it. It will do the same to the extra flesh that grows in the roots of the pterygia.[1]

QUESTION TWO: Double vision (diplopia) has how many causes?

ANSWER: This is recorded in Ibn Sīnā's *Ṭabīʿiyyāt al-shifāʾ*, where he says: There are four causes of double vision. First, the twisting of the mechanism conveying the impression (blurred shape) [of the object seen], which is in the lens, **[38b]** to the junction of the two [optic] nerves. The two impressions do not line up correctly at the same place [in the eye]. Instead, each ends at a part of the visual spirit arranged there by itself because the two lines (i.e., visual rays) of the two impressions did not penetrate in such a way as to meet near the junction of the two [optic] nerves. Therefore, a separate image from each impression that penetrates the lense has to be imprinted separately on part of the visual spirit. Thus, it seems as if there are two images of two separate things on the exterior because the two lines (visual rays) that come out from them to the center of the lens (i.e., two lenses) did not unite while penetrating the two [optic] nerves. Second, the movement of the visual spirit and its oscillations to the right and left, so that the perceptive part goes beyond its center that is traced for it during the imprinting and goes in a disturbed undulating manner in the direction of the lens. Then, the apparition and the image are traced on it (the center) before the junction

---

[1] Cf. Gunther, *Dioscorides*, p. 240; Dubler, *Materia Médica*, II, 240–41. Cf. Ibn Wāfid, p. 203 (Arabic) and p. 263 (Spanish), who says: "If the licorice root is dried, peeled, and cooked and used in a dressing, it is useful for someone who is *dākhis* (suffering from felon, i.e., small abcesses or boils; or whitlow, i.e., sores under or near the nail of a finger or toe) and if it is used copiously it is useful for pterygia which appears in the eyes."

of the two conical forms, and one sees two impressions.[2] This is like the impression traced by the sun on stagnant still water just once, but traced by it on wavy water repeatedly. Third, a disturbance of the movement of the internal spirit, which is behind the junction, to the front and back so that there are two movements in the opposite direction: a movement toward a joint perception and a movement toward the meeting of the two [optic] nerves. Thus, the picture of what is perceived is carried to the two of them another time before what it led to the joint perception disappears. It is as if while what led the picture to the joint perception, part [of the picture] returns and precedes what the visual force conveys, **[39a]** and that is because of the speed of the movement. Thus, for example, it (the part) can be traced in the conveying spirit as a picture. Then it gives it (the picture) to the joint perception. Everything that is traced is fixed for a time until it disappears. When the first receptive thing from the [visual] spirit disappears from its (i.e., the spirit's) center because of a disturbance of its movement, another part follows it and is received before the disappearance of the first. Then, because of the disturbance, the spirit moves to an advanced part that was in the path of what is seen. One perceives it and then it disappears, but the picture does not disappear at once. Indeed, it stays there and [goes] to another part that also receives the picture in the same way. One perceives the picture after the first part and the cause is the disturbance. Fourth, a

[2] According to the Galenic view, vision occurred through a ray that went from the eye to the object and, either by touching the object or compressing the intermediate air, sent an impression of the object to the brain. The rays formed a cone in the eye. See, e.g., A.I. Sabra, "The Scientific Enterprise," in Bernard Lewis, ed., *Islam and the Arab World* (New York: Alfred Knopf, 1976), p. 188. Ḥunayn ibn Isḥāq explains in the following manner why one does not see an object double: "For since each perceived object is seen only by the glances proceeding from the two pupils; and since these looks are like rectilineal lines going straight forward, in the manner in which the rays of the sun penetrate through a window into a house; and since the origin of those lines is united and compressed, whilst their end is broad and separated; and since their general shape in each eye is conical, i.e., the shape of pine-cones, it is an unavoidable necessity that the two central lines of these two (conical) shapes known as axes should be in the same position and that their course should run on the same plane, until the perceived object reaches him (the observer) at the same spot in his eye; [if this were not so, the two lines would not both reach him at the same spot in his eye]. In the same way it is equally necessary for the lines around each of the two axes to be in a position which is alike in both eyes; (finally) the position of the entire conus formed by the lines coming out of one of the eyes must be similar to the position of the entire conus formed by the lines coming out of the other eye. The inevitable consequence of this state of affairs is that the origin of the glances proceding from the two pupiles is the same, and that their course lies along the same flat plane." See Max Meyerhof, ed. and trans., *The Book of the Ten Treatises on the Eye Ascribed to Hunain Ibn Is-Hāq* (Cairo: Government Press, 1928), pp. 25–26.

disturbance of a movement that occurs to the ocular hole. The ocular membrane[3] easily adjusts in shape, expanding to accomodate the hole. Sometimes the hole narrows to the exterior and sometimes to the interior in normal fashion or in some other way. {When it is pushed to the exterior, this results from a compression occurring in it and the expansion of the ocular hole.}[4] When it is pushed to the interior, it follows a conjunction that occurs with it. If it happens that the hole narrows, you see [the thing] larger. If it expands, you see the thing smaller. If it happens that the hole inclines in a certain direction, one sees [the thing] in another place. It is as if what is seen first is different from what is seen second. This is especially so if another image appears before the disappearance of the first.[5]

QUESTION THREE: Which disease of the eye is cured by sprinkling old worn sugar cane on it?

ANSWER: This is recorded in *al-Malakī*, where the author says: If old worn sugar cane is finely pulverized and sprinkled on **[39b]** the eye, it is useful against leucoma of the cornea.[6]

QUESTION FOUR: How many things are harmful to the vision and what are they?

ANSWER: This is recorded in the third book of *al-Qānūn*, where the author says: There are three. First, [certain] actions and movements. Second, [certain] foods. And third, the state of the foods. As for actions, examples are excessive coitus, protracted gazing at shiny things, excessively reading fine script with concentration. But if these things are done in moderation, they are beneficial. The same is true of activities requiring detailed work, sleeping on a full stomach and [right after] dinner. Indeed, it is necessary for anyone with poor vision to wait until his food is digested before sleeping, for sleeping on a full stomach will harm the vision. Everything that dries the nature is also harmful, as is everything that makes the blood turbid, namely, salty, acrid, and sweet things. As for vomiting, it can be helpful when it purifies the stomach but harmful when it activates substances in the brain and pushes them to the vision. If vomiting is inevitable, it is necessary that it occur after

---

3 *Ṭabaqa*: literally layer or membrane. See below n. 13.

4 The sentence in braces is found in the *Ṭabīʿiyyāt* but not in al-Sulamī. Its deletion from the latter was no doubt a copyist's error.

5 Ibn Sīnā, *Ṭabīʿiyyāt*, VI (*al-Nafs*), 134–38.

6 *Al-Malakī*, II, 285, which states that old worn sugar cane is that which is found in old ceilings.

eating and be done gently. Taking a bath, excessive sleep, a lot of crying, many phlebotomies, and especially continuous cupping are harmful. As for harmful foods, they are the rotten, the salty, the acrid, what injures the cardia, eating leeks,[7] onions,[8] garlic, melissa,[9] olives,[10] cabbage, dill, and lentils.[11] As for the state of the foods used, if they are eaten, one should be wary of their decay and large amount of vapor.[12]

QUESTION FIVE: If you see that the eye is black, how **[40a]** do you know if it is from the membranes?[13]

ANSWER: This is recorded in *al-Qānūn*. As for blackness because of moistness, the vision at night is less because of the need to stare and the moving of the substance (moistness) to the exterior. If the substance is abundant, it is more difficult to see than if it is less. As for blackness because of the membranes, it makes the vision stronger.[14]

QUESTION SIX: How does one know if the eye is blue because of a small amount of albuminoid (aqueous) humor, and what is the cause of this?

ANSWER: In this case, one has more vision at night and in darkness than during the day because of the movement caused by the small amount of substance (humor). The movement distracts it from making things clear. Such a movement makes one unable to see things clearly, like the inability to see clearly what is in the dark.[15]

QUESTION SEVEN: What are the general principles for treating eye diseases?

ANSWER: When the diseases are a mixture of substances, a simple mixture, compounded, or separation of connection [of tissue], the

---

7 *Kurrāth*: al-Kindī, pp. 323–24; al-Samarqandī, p. 234.

8 *Baṣal*: al-Samarqandī, pp. 29, 172, 214.

9 *Bādarūj*: *Tuḥfa*, pp. 33–34.

10 *Zaytūn*: *EI*[2], *s.v.* "Zaytūn" (Penelope C. Johnstone).

11 *ʿAdas*: al-Kindī, p. 302; al-Samarqandī, p. 184.

12 *Al-Qānūn*, II, 112; J. Hirschberg and J. Lippert, trans., *Die Augenheilkunde des Ibn Sina* (Leipzig: Verlag von Velt & Comp., 1902), pp. 26–27. Cf. ʿAlī ibn ʿĪsā, *Tadhkira*, pp. 314–16. See n. 18 below for full reference.

13 *Ṭabaqāt*, literally layers or membranes, usually translated as tunics (χιτών). The eye was believed to be composed of as many as seven of these: the retina, choroïd, sclerotic, the one covering the external half of the lense (arachnoïd), uvea (iris), cornea, and conjunctiva. See Meyerhof, ed. and trans., *Ten Treatises on the Eye*, pp. 4–5, 10–12, which include two illustrations.

14 *Al-Qānūn*, II, 131; Hirschberg and Lippert, trans., *Augenheilkunde*, pp. 98–99.

15 *Al-Qānūn*, II, 131; Hirschberg and Lippert, trans., *Augenheilkunde*, p. 98.

treatment of the eye is either purging it–and this includes dealing with inflamations–or changing the mixture, restoring the shape, as with a protruding eyeball, cicatrizing, or mending. The eye rids itself of substances by draining them off or by having them seep away. Being drained of them is better for the body if it is plethoric. As for seeping them away with tear-causing medications or changing the mixture, this is done with special medications. As for the separation of connection, it is treated with the medication that dries slightly but does not burn at all.[16]

QUESTION EIGHT: **[40b]** If a pain in the eye is accompanied by a fierce headache, which is treated first?

ANSWER: The headache is treated first. The eye is not treated until you get rid of it. If purging, purifying, and good treatment are of no help, you should know that there is a bad mixture or a bad substance concealed in the membranes, and it corrupts the nourishment coming to them, or there is a weakness in the brain or in a place from which [bad] substances are discharged to the eye.[17]

QUESTION NINE: What part of the eye, if afflicted by a certain disease, makes the eye water so it does not see?

ANSWER: This is recorded in the third treatise of *al-Tadhkira*, where the author says: If the triangular muscle that is at the opening of the optic nerve contracts, it (the nerve) pulls the eye and binds it.[18]

QUESTION TEN: How many causes are there of night-blindness?

ANSWER: Five causes as recorded in the third treatise of *al-Tadhkira*: moisture occurring in the albuminoid humor, thickening of the psychic spirit, ice-like humor (or crystalline lense) and its turbidity, prolonged exposure to the sun, and vapor from the stomach.[19]

---

[16] *Al-Qānūn*, II, 111; Hirschberg and Lippert, trans., *Augenheilkunde*, pp. 21–22.

[17] *Al-Qānūn*, II, 112; Hirschberg and Lippert, trans., *Augenheilkunde*, p. 24.

[18] This answer is from ʿAlī ibn ʿĪsā al-Kaḥḥāl's (d. after 400/1010) *Tadhkirat al-kaḥḥālīn* ["Promptuary for Oculists"]. See the edition by Ghawth Muḥyī l-Dīn al-Qādirī (Hyderabad: Dāʾirat al-Maʿārif al-ʿUthmāniyya, 1964), p. 307. An English translation was made by C.A. Wood entitled *Memorandum Book of a Tenth-Century Oculist* (Chicago: Northwestern University Press, 1936), primarily from the German translation by J. Hirschberg *et al.* called *ʿAlī bin-ʿĪsā: Errinerungsbuch für Augenärzte* (Leipzig, 1904). Wood did not know Arabic, but consulted Max Meyerhof, who compared his translation with an Arabic MS and together they concluded that he had captured the "essence" of the *Tadhkira*; cf. p. 208. On Ibn ʿĪsā and this work, see *GAL* I, 483, and *S* I, 884–85; *GAS* III, 337–40; Ullmann, *Medizin*, pp. 208–209; *EI*^{2}, *s.v.* "ʿAlī b. ʿĪsā" (E. Mittwoch).

[19] Ibn ʿĪsā, *Tadhkira*, p. 295, gives four primary and one secondary cause. Cf. Wood, *Memorandum Book*, p. 201; Meyerhof, *Ten Treatises*, p. 73.

QUESTION ELEVEN: How many diseases are there of the albuminoid humor?

ANSWER: Seven. They are change in color, [total] dryness, partial dryness, shrinking, enlarging, moistening, and thickening.[20]

QUESTION TWELVE: How many ways does **[41a]** the albuminoid humor change color?

ANSWER: Three. [First], if all of it changes, one sees the whole object in the same color into which it (the albuminoid humor) has changed. Second, it can change at certain times because of the vapors arising to it from the stomach. Then you see the objects according to the vapors. Third, if some of it (the albuminoid humor) has changed, then one sees in front of him objects similar in color and shape to the [colored] parts of the humor.[21]

QUESTION THIRTEEN: How many diseases are characteristic of the eyelids?

ANSWER: Twelve (*sic*): scabies, chalazion, lithiasis, adhesion [to the eye], contraction of the eyelids, sties, superfluous lashes, ingrown lashes, chemosis, lippitude of the eyelids, and papilloma.[22]

QUESTION FOURTEEN: From how many causes can a disease cause one to see at night but not see during the day?

ANSWER: Three: excessive dryness of the visual vital spirit, or from its scarcity and weakness or excessive dissolution.[23]

QUESTION FIFTEEN: What is the difference between dilation [of the pupil] and dispersion [of light (i.e., visual spirit)]?

ANSWER: This is recorded in *al-Tadhkira.* Dilation occurs in the uveal [membrane] or the optic nerve while dispersion occurs in the light (i.e., is a dispersion of light rays). Dilation is a disease while dispersion is a symptom.[24]

---

[20] Ibn ʿĪsā, *Tadhkira*, p. 285. Cf. Wood, *Memorandum Book*, p. 195; Meyerhof, *Ten Treatises*, pp. 49–52.

[21] Ibn ʿĪsā, *Tadhkira*, pp. 286–87. Cf. Wood, *Memorandum Book*, p. 196; Meyerhof, *Ten Treatises*, pp. 50–51.

[22] Ibn ʿĪsā, *Tadhkira*, gives eleven, pp. 75–76. Cf. Wood, *Memorandum Book*, pp. 84–85; Meyerhof, *Ten Treatises*, pp. 58–60.

[23] Ibn ʿĪsā, *Tadhkira*, p. 297. Cf. Wood, *Memorandum Book*, p. 202.

[24] Ibn ʿĪsā, *Tadhkira*, pp. 302–303. Cf. Wood, *Memorandum Book*, p. 205; Meyerhof, *Ten Treatises*, p. 48.

QUESTION SIXTEEN: How many reasons are there for using sticky moist things in the eye?

ANSWER: This is recorded in *al-Tadhkira*. Four: first, because they are non-burning; **[41b]** second, because they stick to the rawness resulting from sharpness (i.e., of the albuminoid humor flowing to the eye) and wash it; third, because they stay in the eye longer than the watery applications; and fourth, because the eye is a sensitive organ. Most of the medications used to treat it are gritty. If anything rough is put on it, its harmfulness is greatly felt. So doctors choose to mix something with it that softens its rawness and sooths it: like egg white, water of fenugreek, watery (tree) gums, tragacanth, and so forth.[25]

QUESTION SEVENTEEN: What is the difference between sclerophthalmia occurring in the eyelid and a thickness?

ANSWER: This is recorded in *al-Tadhkira*. Sclerophthalmia is not accompanied by an inflamation. It is a stiffness that occurs in the eyelid. This occurs in one or both eyelids. Coldness and dryness cause it. Thickness is accompanied by an inflamation. It occurs in both eyelids together. A cold, moist, viscous substance causes it.[26]

QUESTION EIGHTEEN: What is the difference between a protrusion (or prolapse) of the iris (proptoma) and pimples occurring on the cornea?

ANSWER: This is recorded in *al-Tadhkira*. It is necessary to see what color the iris is. Then compare that color to [that of] the illness. If it is not of the same color, you will know {that it is a pimple. Then look also at the pupil itself. If it is small[er than normal] or distorted from its [normal] round shape, you will know}[27] that it is a protrusion on the iris. If you do not see anything like this, it is a pimple. If it (i.e., the color of the protrusion) is the same as the color of the iris, then look at the root of the protruding thing and at the pimple itself. If you see [at] the root of the protruding thing a white trace, you will know that the white thing is a puncture of the cornea and the protruding thing [springs] from the iris. If you do not see anything like this, **[42a]** then it is a pimple.[28]

---

[25] Ibn 'Īsā, *Tadhkira*, p. 48. Cf. Wood, *Memorandum Book*, pp. 33–34.

[26] Ibn 'Īsā, *Tadhkira*, p. 125. Cf. Wood, *Memorandum Book*, pp. 108–109.

[27] The words within braces are lacking from al-Sulamī but are found in *al-Tadhkira*. Clearly, they were mistakenly left out by a copyist, since without them this answer would make no sense.

[28] Ibn 'Īsā, *Tadhkira*, p. 254. Cf. Wood, *Memorandum Book*, pp. 175–76; Meyerhof, *Ten Treatises*, p. 67.

QUESTION NINETEEN: How does one distinguish between a protrusion of the cornea (staphyloma) and a pimple occurring on it?

ANSWER: As for the protrusion, it is hard and stiff. If you touch it with a probe, it will not be depressed because of its hardness. As for pimples, lachrymation and throbbing accompany them and the white [of the eye] becomes red.[29]

QUESTION TWENTY: At what point during an illness do you use aromatic powder?

ANSWER: This is recorded in *al-Tadhkira.* Beware of using aromatic powders at the beginning of ophthalmia or ulcers, because they are extremely harmful unless you are confident of the purity of the body and the head. Then, the author said: At the beginning and at the increase [of an illness], be careful of using a powder in which there is sarcocolla, for it will bring great harm to the patient.[30]

---

[29] Ibn 'Īsā, *Tadhkira*, p. 242. Cf. Wood, *Memorandum Book*, p. 168; Meyerhof, *Ten Treatises*, pp. 66–67.

[30] Ibn 'Īsā, *Tadhkira*, pp. 167–68. Cf. Wood, *Memorandum Book*, pp. 130–31.

CHAPTER EIGHT

ON WHAT A SURGEON SHOULD BE ASKED, COMPRISING TWENTY QUESTIONS

QUESTION ONE: How many bones are in the body?

ANSWER: This is recorded in *al-Qānūn* and Ibn Jumayʿ[1] had [also] recorded it. According to the latter's classification, there are 246 (*sic*) bones. As he specifies, the skull is 2 bones, what is below it are 5, *couples joug*[2] are 4, the upper jawbones are 12, the nose is 2, the teeth are 32, the lower jawbones are 2,[3] the vertebrae of the **[42b]** spinal column are 30, the ribs are 24, the sternum is 7, the two shoulder blades are 2, the two collarbones are 2, the two upper arms are 2, the two forearms are 4, the two wrists are 16, the two metacarpals are 8, the fingers are 30, the pubic region is 2, the two thighs are 2, the two legs are 4, and the two feet are 52. This is what Ibn Jumayʿ says. As for the author of *al-Qānūn*, he says that the number of bones is 248 except the condyle and the bone that resembles the letter *lām* (ل).[4] Ibn Jumayʿ says: The two remaining bones are the upper parts of the shoulders.

QUESTION TWO: How many muscles are in the body?

ANSWER: Five hundred and twenty-nine muscles. Specifically, the face has 9, the two eyes have 24, the lower jawbone (sic) has 12, the two jawbones have 14, the head has 23, the windpipe has 4, the larynx has 16, the bone resembling the letter *lām* has 6, the tongue has 9, the pharynx

---

[1] On Abū l-Makārim Hibat Allāh ibn Jumayʿ al-Isrāʾīlī (d. 594/1198), see *GAL* I, 489, and *S* I, 892; Dietrich, *Medicinalia*, pp. 107–110, 214–15; Ullmann, *Medizin*, p. 164, index; Fähndrich, *Treatise to Ṣalāḥ ad-Dīn*, p. 1–3. For this answer, see *al-Qānūn*, I, 29–39; P. de Koning, ed. and trans., *Trois traités de'anatomie arabes* (Leiden: E.J. Brill, 1903), p. 516; Shah, *Principles*, pp. 54–78.

[2] One of the bones in the head: Koning, *Trois traités*, p. 461 n. 8.

[3] At the beginning of the seventh/thirteenth century, ʿAbd al-Laṭīf al-Baghdādī discovered in Egypt that the lower jaw consisted of one piece, not two as Galen and, therefore, Muslim and other Middle Eastern doctors had taught. His discovery was never incorporated, however, into subsequent Islamic medical literature. Galen remained supreme. See Ullmann, *Islamic Medicine*, p. 71.

[4] Ibn Sīnā means the Greek letter *lamda* (Λ) and not the Arabic letter *lām*. According to Koning, this bone is the *os lingual* or *os hyoïde*, and he adds: "Le nom d'os lamdoïde ne convient pas à l'os lingual (os hyoïde) de l'homme, mais à celui de certains animaux. . . ."; *Trois traités*, p. 453 n. 4. On the number of bones in the body, cf. *ibid.*, pp. 22–23 (al-Rāzī) and 148–51 (*al-Malakī*).

has 2, the neck has 4, the joint between the shoulders and the upper arms has 26, the two elbows have 8, the forearms have 34, the palms have 36, the chest has 107, the spinal column has 48, the stomach has 8, the bladder has 1, the penis has 4, the two testicles have 4, the anus has 4, the hips have 26 for moving the thighs, the thighs have 20 for moving the legs, the legs have 28, and the feet have 52, although some say 55.[5]

[43a] QUESTION THREE: How many cerebral, spinal, and other nerves are in the body?

ANSWER: Thirty-eight pairs and one that is by itself. Specifically, the cerebral nerves are 7 [pairs], the spinal are 31 pairs, and then the one by itself. From the vertebra of the neck there are 8 pairs, from the vertebra of the chest there are 12 pairs, from the vertebra of the small of the back there are 5 pairs, from the bones of the buttocks there are 3 pairs, and from the extremity of the coccyx merges the nerve that is by itself.[6]

QUESTION FOUR: What is the number of veins that are usually bled?

ANSWER: Thirty-three veins. There are twelve in the two hands: the two cephalic veins, the two interior basilic veins, the two basilic veins of the armpits, the two medial arm veins, the two veins of the forearms, and the two *usailims*.[7] There are thirteen in the head and neck: the two veins of the two temples, the two veins behind the two ears, the two veins of the inner corners of the eyes, the two jugular veins, the vein of the crown of the head, the vein of the forehead, the vein at the rear of the head, the vein of the tip of the nose, and the vein under the tongue. This is what the author of *al-Malakī* says. I read in this place a marginal note [which states that] the four veins [of the lips] are comprised of two in the upper and two in the lower lip. There are eight in the two legs: two in the hollow of the knees, two in the two legs, two sciatic veins, and two in the metatarsals of the two feet.[8]

QUESTION FIVE: How many principles **[43b]** must one observe when treating a separation of connection [of tissue] occurring in the soft organs?

---

5 *Al-Malakī*, I, 92–93; Koning, trans., *Trois traités*, pp. 276–79, cf. pp. 26–29 (al-Rāzī), and 518–78 (*al-Qānūn*).

6 *Al-Malakī*, I, 63–67; Koning, trans., *Trois traités*, pp. 153–63, cf. pp. 30–33 (al-Rāzī) and 582–602 (*al-Qānūn*).

7 According to Koning, *Trois traités*, p. 814: "Petite veine salutaire. Veine salvatelle. Partie de la veine basilique, située à la face dorsale de la main et correspondant au quatrième espace intermétacarpien."

8 *Al-Malakī*, II, 460.

ANSWER: This is recorded in *al-Kulliyyāt*. The principles to follow in treatment are three. First, if the cause is stabilized, one must first stop what flows (i.e., the bleeding) and stop its substance (i.e., any discharge) if it (the substance) aggravates it. Second, mending the tear with appropriate medication and diet. Third, preventing decay as much as possible.[9]

QUESTION SIX: How many things keep an ulcer from healing and how does one take steps to prevent each of them?

ANSWER: This is recorded in *al-Kulliyyāt*. Four. [Bad] temperament of the organ, [in which case] one must see to its recovery. Second, bad temperament of the blood going to it, [in which case] one must take steps to promote what generates favorable gastric juice. Third, an abundance of blood that flows to it, [in which case] one takes steps to treat it by purging, using a mild diet, and using exercise if possible. Fourth, the decay of the bone under it and the issue of pus. There is no treatment for this except to heal that bone. Scrape it if the scraping eliminates its decay, or take it and cut it.[10]

QUESTION SEVEN: Which medications should be used for ulcers of the urethra?

ANSWER: This is recorded in the fourth treatise of Galen's *Ḥīlat al-bur'*,[11] where he says: Ulcers of the urethra require an increase in dryness commensurate with the excesive dryness of its (the urethra's) nature. [Dry medication should be used, like] burned paper, burned alum,[12] burned dry pumpkin, and aloe (*ṣabir*). At the beginning, one should use any of them **[44a]** or one like them and it should be sprinkled on the ulcer.

QUESTION EIGHT: What is the condition if a puncture strikes a nerve and what is the method of treatment?

ANSWER: This is recorded in the sixth treatise of Galen's *Ḥīlat al-bur'*, where he says: If a puncture strikes a nerve, it is inevitably highly sensitive so that a pain stronger than that in any other part of the body seizes it. Therefore, it will certainly become inflamed if a subsiding of the pain does not occur and it (the subsiding) prevents the inflamation. This is done by leaving the place of the perforation of the skin the way it is and

[9] *Al-Qānūn*, I, 217–18. Cf. Gruner, *Canon*, pp. 521–22; Shah, *Principles*, p. 415.

[10] *Al-Qānūn*, I, 218–19. Cf. Gruner, *Canon*, p. 524; Shah, *Principles*, p. 417.

[11] On the *Kitāb fī ḥīlat al-bur'* ["Book on the Means of Recovering One's Health"], the Arabic of which has not been published, see *GAS* III, 96–98; Ullmann, *Medizin*, p. 45.

[12] *Shabb*: al-Kindī, pp. 291–92; al-Samarqandī, p. 237.

preventing it from closing so that the pus that oozes from the place of the puncture is expelled. The entire body is cleansed of superfluities by bleeding the vein, if one has the strength to endure it, and of bad mixtures [of humors] with a purging medication. This is what should be done immediately. If the wound is widened, it should be bathed in [edible] oil, in which there are no astringents, after it is heated. It is best if the oil is two or three years old, because it will dissolve more quickly. A medication should be chosen that is composed of gentle compounds, is of moderate heat, and dries without harm like mastic of terebinth, a little of euphorbium,[13] soot, sagapenum, opoponax, asafetida[14] in [people with] firm bodies, and sulphur that has not been exposed to fire. Any of these are mixed with [edible] oil so that they become thick like honey and the wound is dressed with it.[15]

QUESTION NINE: For ulcers of the nerves, is it permissible to use **[44b]** things that loosen or to use hot water?

ANSWER: This is recorded in the sixth treatise of the *Ḥīlat al-bur'*, where the author says: Be careful not to use hot water or loosening medications for ulcers of the nerves.

QUESTION TEN: How many procedures are required for operating on stab (or arrow) wounds?

ANSWER: This is recorded in the sixth treatise of Galen's *Ḥīlat al-bur'*. There are four procedures. This is where he says: Operating on stabs requires four procedures. The first is to sew up the wound. The second is to apply to it only things that expel or pass out from the intestines. The third is to apply an appropriate medication. The fourth is that we should take every precaution, so that no harm will befall the vital organs because of the wound.

QUESTION ELEVEN: If [part of] the intestines comes out and the air makes it cold and then it becomes inflamed, how is it treated?

ANSWER: This is recorded in the sixth treatise of the *Ḥīlat al-bur'*, where the author says: It is necessary to make it warm, so that the gas [in the abdomen] is dissipated from it. Warm it with a sponge [that has been] immersed in hot water, squeezed, and then applied as a compress to it and [administer] a constipating drink. If the drink is heated, the patient will benefit from this, and it will combine its warmth with the strength

13 *Furbiyūn*: al-Kindī, p. 311; al-Samarqandī, p. 226.

14 *Ḥiltīt*: al-Kindī, p. 260. The gum of *anjudān*, Chapter 5 n. 249 above.

15 Cf. al-Rāzī, *al-Ḥāwī*, XII, 182–83.

of the intestines. If the condition remains inflamed and the wound is narrow, it is necessary to cleave the dermis to the extent that is required for the protruding intestines to enter.

QUESTION **[45a]** TWELVE: Is the method of treating ulcers on the width of a muscle like that of those on its length?

ANSWER: This is recorded in Galen's *Ḥīlat al-bur'*, where he says: [If] ulcers occur on the width of a muscle, the skin is widely separated and it is necessary to bring the two sides together more firmly and in a more lasting fashion. Thus, it needs to be sewed up and supported with triangular bandages. Ulcers occurring on the length of a muscle can be brought together by bandaging unless the wound is deep, [in which case] it requires a small amount of sewing up or bandages without sewing up.

QUESTION THIRTEEN: What are the benefits of a phlebotomy?

ANSWER: This is recorded in Galen's *Kitāb al-Faṣd*.[16] There are two kinds. One is the elimination of plethora, and the other is the neutralization of an illness that is caused by a blow, a strong pain, or a weak organ. By means of a phlebotomy, the organs push out (illnesses, superfluities, corruption, etc.).

QUESTION FOURTEEN: What is the method of treating a wound if it occurs in the head and reaches the region of the membrane (pericranium)?

ANSWER: This is recorded in the fourteenth treatise of *al-Malakī*, where the author says: When a wound occurs in the head and reaches the regions of the brain and the membrane, it is not necessary to hasten with medications that heal and mend. If you do that, you will bring injury to the patient because the brain will become inflamed, **[45b]** the mind will become confused, and convulsions will occur. But placing in the wound a piece of wool that has been soaked in [edible] oil for three days will take care of the inflamation and convulsions. After this, you should use ointments and mending aromatic powders, like the powders made from myrrh, aloe (*ṣabir*), frankincense, black salve,[17] and the like.[18]

QUESTION FIFTEEN: What is the method of treating an ulcer accompanied by a broken bone?

[16] On this work ["Book on Phlebotomy"], the Arabic of which has not been published, see *GAS* III, 115–16; and Ullmann, *Medizin*, p. 59. On the phlebotomist, see *EI*^{2}, *Supplement*, *s.v.* "Faṣṣād, Ḥadjdjām" (M.A.J. Beg).

[17] *Al-Marham al-aswad*, probably a mistake for *al-marham al-usrub* (salve of black lead). *Al-Marham al-abyaḍ* is white lead. Al-Rāzī, *al-Murshid*, p. 205.

[18] *Al-Malakī*, II, 217–18.

ANSWER: This is recorded in the fourteenth treatise of *al-Malakī*, where the author says: When an ulcer is accompanied by a broken bone, treat the bone with what one treats the ulcer, [that is], with the strong dressing one uses to set broken bones. If the wound (sic) occurs in the head and the skull is broken but the membrane is not damaged, one must dress the bones with round Aristolochia (see Chapter 5 n. 185) that is fine, powdery, and kneaded with water. This exposes the bone and it should be treated after this with myrrh and struthion[19] in equal parts pounded, sifted, and kneaded in honey and cooked syrup so that they congeal, and then smear it on a gauze tampon and use it in ointments.[20]

QUESTION SIXTEEN: What is the method of treating ulcers if there is a bone beneath them that has decayed, and what is the symptom of this?

ANSWER: This is recorded in *al-Malakī*. As for its symptom, if you notice that the ulcer sometimes heals and returns, and then it opens and pus flows from it and if you insert the tip of a probe into the ulcer and feel a rustling sound, then when you find this to be the case you must apply to it a fiery ointment **[46a]** to consume the dead flesh. If you do this and the place becomes like a scab or like loose flesh, then [soak it] with lukewarm ghee until the burned flesh falls away and the bone is exposed. When the bone becomes visible to you and is possible to be cut, then cut it. Otherwise, [if you do not do this, soak it] again with lukewarm ghee until it decays and falls away. It should then be treated for a day with an ointment of verdigris[21] and for a day with worn cotton until the flesh grows and heals.[22]

QUESTION SEVENTEEN: How do you remove a barb or arrowhead that has entered one of the organs and is in a place from which it cannot be extracted with an iron tool?[23]

ANSWER: This is recorded in *al-Malakī*. One must place on the spot where it entered round Aristolochia that is fine, powdery, and kneaded with gum ammoniac. This should be applied for several days. Or, one could obtain the roots of the moist Persian reed,[24] grind it to a powder, mix it with honey, and apply it to the spot. Or, one could obtain

19 *Kundus*: al-Kindī, p. 328; al-Samarqandī, p. 217.

20 *Al-Malakī*, II, 218.

21 *Zinjār*: al-Samarqandī, pp. 171, 234.

22 *Al-Malakī*, II, 218.

23 Cf. K.K. Thakral, "Techniques for Extraction of Foreign Bodies from War Wounds in Medieval India," *Indian Journal of the History of Science* 16i (1981), 11–16.

24 *Al-Qaṣab al-fārisī*: Maimonides, no. 329; Dozy, II, 352.

Nabatean resin[25] and pitch and melt them and mix them with myosote[26] as a fine powder. It will attract the object and extract it.

QUESTION EIGHTEEN: What are the separations of connection [of tissue] occurring on an organ called?

ANSWER: This is recorded in *al-Kulliyyāt*. If it occurs on the skin, it is called an abrasion or scratch. If it occurs in the flesh but is not festering, it is called a wound. If it is festering, it is called an ulcer. If it occurs on a bone, it is called a fracture. If it occurs along its length, it is called a fissure. If it occurs along the width of a nerve, it is called a severance. If it occurs **[46b]** along its length and is not multiple, it is called a cleft. But if it is multiple, it is called a laceration. If it occurs at the end of a muscle, it is called a tear, whether it is on a nerve or tendon. If it occurs along the width of a muscle, it is called a clipping. If it occurs along its length, is very deep, and few in number, it is called a crushing. If its elements are numerous, it spreads, and it is very deep, it is called a bruise and severance. Sometimes the terms severance, bruise, and crushing are used for whatever happens in the middle of a muscle, whatever it is. If it occurs in the arteries, it is called *umm al-damm* ("bloody"). If it occurs in the veins, it is called an eruption. If it is along the width, it is called a cutting or separation. If it penetrates along its length, it is called a fissure. If its apertures are open, it is called a puncture. If it is in the membranes and diaphragms, it is called a rupture. If it occurs between two parts of a compound organ and one of them separates from the other without injury to either, it is called a separation and dislocation. If this occurs in a nerve that leaves its place, it is called a disjoining.[27]

QUESTION NINETEEN: How many steps must someone who performs circumcisions consider before and after the circumcision?

ANSWER: This is recorded in Aḥmad ibn 'Alī al-Fārisī's treatise *Fī l-Taṭhīr*,[28] where he says: It is necessary to consider seven steps. First, it is necessary for the body to be cleansed before the circumcision. Second, [one must know] the diet that improves the health of the person who is to be circumcised. Third, [one must know] how to operate and the implements that **[47a]** are used for operating. Fourth, [one must know] the aromatic powders that stop the bleeding. Fifth, [one must know]

---

25 *'Ilk al-anbāṭ*: al-Kindī, p. 306.

26 *Adhān al-fār*: Levey, *Toxicology*, p. 115.

27 *Al-Qānūn*, I, 75–76. Cf. Gruner, *Canon*, pp. 163–64; Shah, *Principles*, pp. 145–46.

28 This work ["On Purification," i.e., circumcision] is unidentified. Indeed, it may not be a title, i.e., "al-Fārisī's treatise on circumcision."

the ointments that are especially effective for mending. Sixth, [one must know] the ointments that cleanse the urethra. And seventh, [one must know] about entering the bath and the time when this must be done.

QUESTION TWENTY: What is the special ointment for the urethra during circumcision, and when is it used?

ANSWER: This is recorded in al-Sūsī's treatise *Fī l-Taṭhīr*.[29] He says: An ointment of unique ingredients is good for the bodies of youths and the bodies of the tender. It is used on the second day after the circumcision. Its formula is one half *raṭl* of rose oil and one quarter *raṭl* of litharge,[30] which is ground up and sifted until it is like kohl. Then it is cooked with the oil until it is like wax that will not stain the hand. Then it is removed from the fire and ten *dirhams* of bleached white wax (see Chapter 5 n. 17) and an *ūqiyya* (one twelfth of a *raṭl*) of cow ghee and ten *dirhams* of burned acacia washed in rose-water, pulverized and sifted, and seven *dirhams* of Socotran aloe are mixed with it and then cooked over a gentle fire and constantly stirred until it becomes like wax and is then removed.

---

29 Al-Sūsī may be the same person as al-Fārisī in the previous question.

30 *Mardāsanj*: al-Samarqandī, p. 235. For the *raṭl* and *dirham* as standards of measure, see *EI*[1], *s.v.* "Raṭl" (A. S. Atiya); *EI*[2], *s.v.* "Dirham" (G.C. Miles); Walter Hinz, *Islamische Masse und Gewichte* (Leiden: E.J. Brill, 1970), pp. 1–8, 27–33.

CHAPTER NINE

ON WHAT THE BONESETTER SHOULD BE ASKED, COMPRISING TWENTY QUESTIONS

QUESTION ONE: Which parts of the body are difficult to be dislocated, which are easy to be dislocated, and which are in between?

ANSWER: This is recorded in **[47b]** the fourth book of *al-Qānūn*, where the author says: It is easy to dislocate such parts as the knee joint because of the pliability of the ligaments. It is also easy to be reset. A shoulder joint is much like this in slender people. It is difficult to dislocate such parts as the joints of the fingers because they will almost always break before being dislocated. An elbow joint is just like this and its return to normal is difficult. As for those in between, they are like the joints of the hip. The most difficult dislocation is when the tips of the small pieces of bone that fasten one bone to another are broken with it. Seldom will it return to its natural state. This usually concerns the apex of the hip, then the apex of the forearm and the two bones of the ankle when there is a break.[1]

QUESTION TWO: What are the symptoms of a dislocation, what are the symptoms of a deviation, and what are the symptoms of a hyperextension of the joint without a dislocation?

ANSWER: A dislocation occurring in the joint [presents] an unusual depression and hollow, like what happens in the joint of the leg. Even more apparent [is what] occurs in the joint of the neck. Comparison will reveal a normal condition, and that by comparing the ill with its healthy counterpart. If you notice that the joint does not move in every direction, it is not a malady associated with slippage [of a joint (subluxation)]. As for the symptoms of a deviation, this is if one sees a depression with a protrusion on the other side, although some movement is possible. As for the symptoms of a hyperextension of the joint without **[48a]** a dislocation, it is as if it were dangling. If you push it in, it returns to its natural place without difficulty. If you leave it, it returns to the accidental shape and there will be a hollow. Sometimes the finger penetrates where there is not much flesh, like the shoulder.[2]

---

[1] *Al-Qānūn*, III, 187.

[2] *Ibid*.

QUESTION THREE: How many kinds of simple skull fractures are there?

ANSWER: Six, recorded in *al-Malakī*, where the author says: A fracture that occurs in the skull can be simple or compound. A simple fracture is one on the head that is apparent and deep, but there is no separation of bone and no part of bone comes out or goes inside. Another is a crack accompanied by broken bone coming out. Another is when the skull is broken into many pieces and the fracture extends as deep as the dura mater. Another is when the broken bone occurs underneath near the dermis. Another is a large crack in the head resulting in the penetration of the bone into the head. Another is the hairline variety. It is a fine crack that cannot be felt and is not noticed, although sometimes it can be fatal.[3]

QUESTION FOUR: What is a comminuted fracture and how many kinds are there?

ANSWER: This is recorded in *al-Malakī*, where the author says: As for a comminuted fracture, it is not a cracked bone but an inward denting in which the bone holds together without coming apart, like what happens to something that is soft like lead or silver **[48b]** when a body harder than it bumps it. There are two kinds [of comminuted fractures]: either the bone is crushed through its entire thickness so that it usually extrudes the pia mater, or the bone of the head is compressed with the surface of the mater which is on the skull [at the place of the wound].[4]

QUESTION FIVE: Which is faster and easier to treat, a sharply defined broken bone or a non-sharply defined broken bone?

ANSWER: This is recorded in *al-Malakī*. The sharply defined is easier because stretching, straightening, and its return to proper form are possible with it but are not possible with the non-sharply defined.[5]

QUESTION SIX: Which mends faster with regard to a broken forearm, a broken radius or a broken ulna, or both [together]?

ANSWER: This is recorded in *al-Malakī*. As for the two breaking together, this is the most difficult to treat and the most harmful, especially if the two are broken at the same position. As for a broken radius, it mends more slowly and is worse. As for the ulna, it is the faster to mend.[6]

---

3 *Al-Malakī*, II, 501–502.
4 *Ibid.*, II, 502.
5 *Ibid.*, II, 505.
6 *Ibid.*, II, 508.

QUESTION SEVEN: What is a dislocation and what is a slippage of a joint (subluxation)?

ANSWER: This is recorded in *al-Malakī*. A dislocation is a departure of the ball of the bone from the socket into which it fits. If the departure is slight and does not go beyond the socket, it is not called a dislocation but a slippage of the joint.[7]

QUESTION EIGHT: What results from a dislocation of the two jawbones if they are left alone and neglected?

ANSWER: **[49a]** The author of *al-Malakī* said: If they are left alone and not reset, bad symptoms result from this, namely, constant fevers and a constant headache. That is because the muscles of the two jawbones, if they change position, are distended and pull with them the muscles of the temples and stretch them. A fierce headache results from this. Moreover, someone in this condition suffers from diarrhea and vomiting two pure biles (yellow and black). He often dies on the tenth day.[8]

QUESTION NINE: In how many directions does a hip joint usually move?

ANSWER: This is recorded in *al-Malakī*. Four. First, it moves from its position to the inside. Second, it moves from its position to the outside. Third, it moves forward. And fourth, [it moves] backward. Movement forward is the least frequent and movement to the inside is the most frequent.[9]

QUESTION TEN: How many are the directions in which dislocations occur in the knee joint?

ANSWER: This is recorded in *al-Malakī*. Three. First, it slips to the inside. Second, [it slips] to the outside. And third, [it slips] backward. It cannot slip forward because the kneecap prevents this.[10]

QUESTION ELEVEN: What must a bonesetter consider?

ANSWER: This is recorded in *al-Qānūn*. The author says: The bonesetter must consider the angle of a broken bone. Then he will find in the direction to which it slants a hump, and in the direction from which it slants **[49b]** a cavity. Frequently, he can determine this by touch. Also,

---

[7] *Ibid.*, II, 510.

[8] *Ibid.*, II, 510–11. Cf. Hippocrates, *Hippocratic Writings*, Adams trans. p. 100.

[9] *Al-Malakī*, II, 514.

[10] Cf. Hippocrates, *Hippocratic Writings*, Adams trans., p. 121; Chadwich *et al.* trans., p. 309.

the pain becomes intense in the direction to which it slants. He must pass his hand over the place of the fracture, in each case passing gently up and down. He must not be deceived with anything that looks like it is straight before a complete recovery, because inflamation can hide considerable crookedness. It is necessary to set quickly what has broken. Indeed, one should set it the day it happens. The longer one waits, the harder it is to set and the damage will be more. This is especially so with bones surrounded by muscles.[11]

QUESTION TWELVE: At what time should splints be used?

ANSWER: This is recorded in *al-Qānūn*. It is after five or more days until the damage is taken care of. Whenever the limb is enlarged, one should delay in setting the splints in place. Frequently, being in a hurry in this causes damage, so in place of [splints] one should bind [the limb] well with bandages and braces. If that is not possible, then splinting is essential, even from the very beginning. It is necessary to bind the splints very tightly with bandages where the break occurred. If necessary, the bandages should be loosened every two days at the beginning, especially if itching occurs. When seven [days] have passed from the time of tightening the bandages, they can be untied and loosened a little every four or five days. But if you can leave the splints [in place] even for twenty days, without possibility of harm, then do not remove them.[12]

[50a] QUESTION THIRTEEN: What is the principle of bonesetting?

ANSWER: This is recorded in *al-Qānūn*. The principle of bonesetting is to extend the limb as much as necessary. But excessive pulling causes spasms and is painful. Fevers occur and it may sometimes cause limpness. This is less harmful with moist bodies because of their suitability for extending. Not extending sufficiently prevents straight and even mending from occurring. This is true for a dislocation or fracture equally. It is also necessary to rest the limb as much as possible or, in cases in which there is no damage or inflamation, to keep [movement] within bearable limits, otherwise use of the limb will be lost. It is also necessary to avoid causing intense pain while extending and pulling in [cases in which] a fracture and dislocation occur together.[13]

QUESTION FOURTEEN: On which bone will callus[14] not grow?

---

[11] *Al-Qānūn*, III, 200.

[12] *Ibid.*, III, 203.

[13] *Ibid.*, III, 198.

[14] *Dashbad*. According to Dozy, I, 443, *dashbadh* is a bony substance that surgeons apply to a fracture in order to stop the break.

ANSWER: This is recorded in the fourth book of *al-Qānūn*, "On the Fundamentals of Bonesetting and Bandaging." The author says: The aim of most bonesetting is to make callus occur, except in cases involving the bones of the head, because callus will not grow on them.[15]

QUESTION FIFTEEN: What is the binding if the fracture is along the length and is it like the binding if the fracture is across the width or not?

ANSWER: This is recorded in the fourth book of *al-Qānūn*, where the author says: As for a fracture along the length, it suffices to bind the limb very strongly, more so than for other fractures, and it should be squeezed. As for a fracture that is **[50b]** across the width, it is necessary to set the two bones in line as much as possible. Check this with regard to the position of the undamaged parts, and whether or not the damaged part of this bone matches the same spot on the other bone. Then set it and check for splinters, protrusions, and gaps.[16]

QUESTION SIXTEEN: What are the things that harden the callus?

ANSWER: This is recorded in *al-Qānūn*. They are costive and gentle bath aromatics,[17] and dressings similar to them, like cooked myrtle and its oil, an embrocation from the juice of myrtle leaves and seeds, cooked Egyptian mitosa,[18] and the cooked roots of the elm and its cooked leaves. This makes it cohesive and firm. A dressing made with mungo bean, especially with saffron and myrrh, kneaded with syrup of grand basil, is extremely good. The rind of the spathe[19] of the palm tree is also good.[20]

QUESTION SEVENTEEN: Is the mending period of all limbs the same or different? If it is different, what are some examples?

ANSWER: This is recorded in *al-Qānūn*. The mending period is different. For example, the nose mends in ten days, the rib in twenty days, the arm in approximately thirty or forty days, and the thigh in fifty days or sometimes as long as three or four months. Sometimes the forearm mends in twenty-eight days. This is mentioned **[51a]** in the chapter on the fracture of the forearm.[21]

QUESTION EIGHTEEN: What makes bonesetting difficult?

---

15 *Al-Qānūn*, III, 198.

16 *Ibid.*, III, 199.

17 *Nuṭūlāt*: al-Samarqandī, p. 242.

18 *Qarẓ*: Lane, *Lexicon*, I.7, 2518. Cf. al-Kindī, p. 314; Steingass, *qarṭ*, p. 965.

19 *Ṭal'*: Hava, p. 436; Steingass, p. 818.

20 *Al-Qānūn*, III, 205.

21 *Ibid.*, III, 197–98, 215.

ANSWER: Frequently inspecting or frequently untying and retying the bandages, or being in a hurry to move it, or a small amount of viscous blood in the body, or a small amount of blood in general. Therefore, the mending period of the bones of people who are cool or convalescents is shorter.

QUESTION NINETEEN: What do you say about a fractured heel?

ANSWER: This is recorded in *al-Qānūn*. It is difficult to fracture a heel, and it is hard to treat it. It is usually fractured when a person falls from a high place. Sometimes a large bruise occurs with blood flowing to the interior of the muscles, congealing there, and leading to gruesome symptoms. If the heel mends, walking on it is painful. If the heel does not mend properly, it is no longer useful.[22]

QUESTION TWENTY: What is the placement of the heel and what use does it have?

ANSWER: This is recorded in *al-Qānūn*. It is placed under the ankle. It is hard and round in the back in order to resist striking and damage. The bottom is smooth, so that one can walk straight and the foot fits the spot stood upon. Its [weight bearing] capacity is great in order to bear the body. It is in the shape of an elongated triangle and becomes increasingly narrow **[51b]** until it ends and disappears at the hollow of the sole, so that the hollow is gradually deepened from the back to the middle.[23]

---

22 *Ibid.*, III, 217.

23 *Ibid.*, I, 39. Cf. Shah, *Principles*, p. 78.

CHAPTER TEN

ON THE FUNDAMENTALS OF THIS ART, COMPRISING TWENTY QUESTIONS

QUESTION ONE: What is the argument of someone who says that the number of elements is not more than one?

ANSWER: This is recorded in Ibn Sīnā's *al-Shifā'*. When we look at natural things, [we see that] one changes to another. Everything that changes has something constant in it which, during the process of change, is that which changes from one state to another. From this it follows that all natural bodies must retain something in common. This is its (i.e., the one) element.[1]

QUESTION TWO: What is the argument of those who say that the element is fire?

ANSWER: This is recorded in *al-Shifā'*. They are of the opinion that fire is a great essence. They have contempt for the size of the earth and the water and air within it. Indeed, for them the radiant skies and the shining planets are all of the nature of fire. They have concluded that the mass of the greatest amount is most deserving to be an element. In particular, there is no purer body in its nature than fire. Heat is spread throughout the universe, and what is air but fire made languid by the coldness of steam? What is steam but dissolved water? **[52a]** What is water but condensed fire and dense air? Even if coldness has an element with which it is formed, and coldness is not a non-essential matter, there is among the elements something cold and its coldness is commensurate to the strength of the heat of fire.[2]

QUESTION THREE: What is the argument of those who say that the element is one, that is, water?

ANSWER: This is recorded in *al-Shifā'*. They say that the captivity of moisture is more lasting in air than it is in water, and that is because its (i.e., air's) compliance with that captivity is more intense. What is water but condensed air? That which is condensed is closer to dryness than it is to rarification. As for earth, it is the result of strong condensation. For example, we see it in the congealing of flowing liquid (lava?) as stones.

---

1 Ibn Sīnā, *Ṭabī'iyyāt*, II (*al-Samā' wa-l-'ālam*, etc.), 86.

2 *Ibid.*, p. 87.

As for fire, it is nothing but air heated to such an intensity that it craves the heights.[3]

QUESTION FOUR: What is the argument of someone who says that the elements of bodies are two, fire and earth?

ANSWER: This is recorded in Ibn Sīnā's *al-Shifā'*. They say that all of the elements eventually change into these two materials. These two materials do not change into any elements other than themselves, and thus are the two [ultimate] elements. Therefore, they are the highest forms of lightness and heaviness. The other two elements fall short of them. And because there are only two elements in which there is movement, the more dominant of the two is the [primal] element. In comparison with others, fire and earth are the most dominant. Moreover, air is **[52b]** congealed languid fire that is burdened with evaporated water. Water is dissolved liquid earth mixed with the nature of fire. It is lighter than earth.[4]

QUESTION FIVE: What is the argument of someone who says that the two elements are earth and water?

ANSWER: They are of the opinion that the compounds (elements) need wetness and dryness. They need wetness in order to take shape and then need dryness to preserve their shape. Wetness is easy to acquire and easy to remove. But dryness is difficult to acquire and difficult to remove. If dryness blends with wetness, the compound (element) acquires from the wetness good shapeability and from dryness strong preservation of it. Dryness and wetness are visible as none other than earth and water.[5]

QUESTION SIX: What is it that, when taken into account, makes it evident that the four elements are formed from each other?

ANSWER: This is recorded in Ibn Sīnā's *al-Shifā'*, where he says: A reflective individual will find that the plants and animals found on the earth are derived from earth, water, and air and their creation is completed by the fusion of a ripening agent (fire). Earth benefits an organism by holding it together and preserving its shape and delineating it. Water benefits an organism by lending it ease of creation and shapeability. The essence of the water, after it flows, is maintained by mixing with the earth, and the essence of the earth keeps it from breaking up while mixing with water. Air and fire **[53a]** vitiate the purity of these two but

[3] *Ibid.*, p. 88.
[4] *Ibid.*
[5] *Ibid.*, p. 89.

complement them in moderate mixtures. Air rarifies and helps to create openings and pores. Fire matures, cooks, and brings things together. Thus, it is evident that [the four elements] are formed from each other.[6]

QUESTION SEVEN: What is temperament?

ANSWER: This is recorded in *al-Qānūn*, where he says: Temperament is a condition resulting from the interaction of opposing qualities found in elements of minute particles, so that they will have the most contact with each other. When their forces interact with each other, a similar condition occurs in all of them, and this is the temperament.[7]

QUESTION EIGHT: What is ripening? Are there different kinds or not?

ANSWER: This is recorded in *al-Shifā'*. Ripening is a transformation of the heat in a moist body to conform with the intended goal. There are different kinds, namely, the ripening of the genre of the thing, the ripening of food [in the stomach], and the ripening of excess [in the body]. It can also be said that what is induced artificially is [a kind of] ripening. As for the ripening of the genre of the thing, it is like the ripening of fruit. The cause of this ripening is found in the essence of the ripe thing. It transforms its moisture to a sustenance conforming to the intended goal of its existence. This only happens so it can recreate itself. As for the ripening of food, it does not occur like the ripening of the genre of the thing. This is because the ripening of food corrupts the essence of the food and changes it to the natural form of the essence of what is nourished. **[53b]** The cause of this ripening is not found in the essence of what matures. Rather, it is in the essence of what it changes into. But it is a transformation from the heat with the moisture in conformity with the intended goal, which is a benefit in exchange for what is dissolved. The special name for this ripening is "digestion." As for the ripening of excess in itself, that is, by which there is no benefit regarding nourishment, it is distinguished from the first two types. This ripening is a transformation of the moisture into a sustenance and temperament. The repelling of the moisture facilitates it (the ripening) either by thickening its sustenance, if what hinders its repulsion is its excessive flow and thinness, or by thinning it, if what hinders [its repulsion] is its excessive thickness, or by cutting it to pieces, if what hinders [its repulsion] is [too strong] for its coming together.[8]

---

6 *Ibid.*, p. 189.

7 *Al-Qānūn*, I, 6. Cf. Gruner, *Canon*, p. 57; Shah, *Principles*, p. 24. On temperament, see Dols, *Medieval Islamic Medicine*, pp. 13–16; Ullmann, *Islamic Medicine*, p. 57.

8 Ibn Sīnā, *Ṭabīʿiyyāt*, II (*al-Samā' wa-l-ʿālam*), 223–24.

QUESTION NINE: What is the reason that Fusṭāṭ[9] has so little rain but much dampness?

ANSWER: This is recorded in the *Kitāb al-Najāt fī l-masā'il.*[10] They say that steam escapes if it occurs in places devoid of what confines steam, encompasses it, and condenses it. Then it goes beyond to another place until it encounters what confines and encompasses it. If this place is surrounded by mountains and its land gives off a lot of steam because the heat of the sun suits it to doing so, then when the sun sets it becomes cold and at night the steam is transformed into plentiful dew. Or, the place can lack steam because it is not suited to this. In places with a lot of steam and mountains, their steam is confined until it is condensed, thus producing much rain. To the north of Fusṭāṭ there are no towering mountains. Most of the steam that flows into it is from south **[54a]** to north from the direction of the Ethiopian sea.[11] Furthermore, the Nile in Egypt covers all of its land and stays there for some time. When it recedes, the remaining water is absorbed by the land, which accepts it because of its long duration on its surface. The steam that rises every day from its land increases with the heat of the sun, and when the sun sets this steam becomes a cloud. It dissipates at night because of its rarefication, delicateness, and lack of condensation. [Therefore,] the author said: This is the reason for the small amount of rainfall and the large amount of dampness.[12]

QUESTION TEN: How many things are completely and perfectly included in the art of medicine?

ANSWER: This is recorded in Qusṭā ibn Lūqā's *al-Madkhal ilā 'ilm al-ṭibb*,[13] where he says: There are ten. First, the study of the fundamentals of the human body. Second, the study of the humors and compositions on which the fundamentals of the human body are based. Third, the study of the number of organs, their nature, and composition. Fourth, the study of their strength and actions. Fifth, the study of the beneficial

[9] On this city just south of Cairo, see *EI* [2], *s.v.* "al-Fusṭāṭ" (J. Jomier).

[10] This work is unidentified.

[11] Apparently the Arabian Sea; see Vladimir Minorsky, trans., *Ḥudūd al-'ālam* (London: Luzac, 1937), p. 145.

[12] Cf. Ibn Riḍwān's description of dew in Egypt, in Dols, *Medieval Islamic Medicine*, pp. 83–85.

[13] On Qusṭā ibn Lūqā (d. early 4th/10th cent.) and this work ["Introduction to the Science of Medicine"], which apparently is lost, see *GAL* I, 204, and *S* I, 365–66; *GAS* III, 270–74; Dietrich, *Medicinalia*, p. 198; Ullmann, *Medizin*, pp. 126–28, index; Dodge, *Fihrist*, II, 694–95; *EI* [2], *s.v.* "Ḳusṭā b. Lūḳā" (D. Hill).

uses for which they were created. Sixth, the study of the preservation of their health. Seventh, the study of what illnesses occur in them and their symptoms. Eighth, the study of the causes of the illnesses occurring in them. Ninth, the study of the symptoms indicating them. And tenth, the study of the curative treatments that expel **[54b]** the illnesses occurring in them.

QUESTION ELEVEN: How many kinds of organs have similar features?

ANSWER: This is recorded in *al-Malakī*. Seven kinds. First, the bones and cartilage. Second, the nerves and tendons. Third, the non-pulsating veins. Fourth, the pulsating veins (i.e., arteries). Fifth, the simple flesh, glands, and fat. Sixth, the skin and membranes. And seventh, the nails and hair.[14]

QUESTION TWELVE: How many actions are necessary for maintaining life?

ANSWER: This is recorded in the *Ṭabīʿiyyāt al-shifāʾ*. Three. The action of nourishing the body, which originates from the natural faculty. The action of nourishing the [vital] spirit and regulating it, which originates from the vital faculty. And the actions of sensation and movement, which originate from the psychic faculty.[15]

QUESTION THIRTEEN: What are the initial cause, antecedent cause, and connecting cause?

ANSWER: This is recorded in ʿAlī ibn Riḍwān's *Sharḥ aghlūqan*.[16] As for the initial cause, it is what has an effect on the body and ceases. The antecedent cause collects in the body as a substance [of an illness] or causes a bad temperament, like an abundance of humors resulting from a plethora of liquids. The connecting cause is called "the holder," like the decay of the humors. It is the reason that one who is seized by a fever has it as long as he does.

[55a] QUESTION FOURTEEN: What is the fifty-fourth aphorism of the fourth treatise of Hippocrates' *al-Fuṣūl*,[17] and what is the meaning of it?

---

14 *Al-Malakī*, I, 48.

15 If this reference is found in a part of *al-Shifāʾ* that has been published, it has eluded me.

16 The *Sharḥ Kitāb Jālīnūs ilā aghlūqan fī l-taʾannī li-shifāʾ al-amrāḍ* ["Commentary on Galen's *Ad Glauconem* on the Retardation of the Healing of Diseases"] has not been published in its Arabic version. See Schacht and Meyerhof, *Controversy*, pp. 41 and 9 (Arabic).

17 This work ["Aphorisms"] is included in Hippocrates, *Hippocratic Writings*, Adams trans., pp. 131–44, Chadwick *et al.* trans., pp. 206–36. See also *GAL* I, 206 (5a), and *S* I, 368; *GAS* III, 28–32; Ullmann, *Medizin*, p. 28.

ANSWER: As for this aphorism, Hippocrates says: Whoever is inflicted by an ardent fever and a persistent dry cough and his aggravation is little, he will hardly ever be thirsty.[18] Galen interpreted this [to mean that] the dry cough might be from a bad abscess that occurs in the respiratory organs, or from a roughness in the throat, or from a slight and delicate moisture flowing in it. If any of these things occur, it will be as if the trachea of the lungs is closed and therefore there is little thirst.

QUESTION FIFTEEN: What is the sixty-fifth aphorism of the fifth treatise of Hippocrates' *al-Fuṣūl*, and what is the meaning of it?

ANSWER: As for this aphorism, the author says: If large malignant abscesses occur, but no inflamation appears with them, then the affliction is great.[19] Galen interpreted this to mean the malignant abscesses occurring at the apexes of the muscles or at their ends, and especially in the muscles in which the nerves are predominant because the apexes of the muscles are connected to the nerves and the tendons grow from their (the muscles') outermost points. He calls this a great affliction because one cannot be sure if the humors that pour into the abscesses because of the pain occurring in the ulcer will invariably flow to it (the muscle). Then the harm will be great.

QUESTION SIXTEEN: How many principles are there **[55b]** by which illnesses of the internal organs can be recognized?

ANSWER: This is recorded in the first treatise of Galen's *Jawāmiʿ al-taʿarruf*,[20] where he says: Six. First, the harm that afflicts the actions [of the organs]. Second, the things that cause to come out and expel. Third, the inflamations that occur. Fourth, pain. Fifth, special symptoms. And sixth, complications in the illness.

QUESTION SEVENTEEN: How many categories of extranormal things occur in the body?

---

[18] In Hippocrates, *Hippocratic Writings*, Adams trans., p. 137, this aphorism is translated as follows: "In whatever case of ardent fever dry coughs of a tickling nature with slight expectoration are long protracted, there is usually not much thirst." In Chadwich *et al.* trans., p. 220, we find: "In fevers of the type of *causus* where there is a frequent dry cough irritating slightly, thirst is not produced."

[19] In *ibid.*, Adams trans., p. 140, the sixty-fifth aphorism bears no resemblance to this. The sixty-sixth reads: "When no swelling appears on severe and bad wounds it is a great evil." In Chadwich *et al.* trans., p. 227, we find: "If swelling does not occur as a result of serious deep wounds, the outlook is very bad."

[20] The identity of this work ["Diagnostic Summaries"] is uncertain. See *GAS* III, 90, 148; Dietrich, *Medicinalia*, p. 198. Ullmann, *Medizin*, pp. 41–42, mentions a book by Galen entitled *Kitāb Taʿarruf ʿilal al-aʿḍāʾ al-bāṭina*.

ANSWER: This is recorded in the second treatise of Galen's *Ḥīlat al-bur'*. Four. First, the action itself in which harm and injury occur. Second, [what occurs] in the structure and shape causing [the illness]. Third, the active cause of this structure and shape. And fourth, the necessary symptom following this shape and structure. Let us designate the structure and shape of the body that harm or hinder the action as a sickness, and call what follows this a symptom, and call the active thing that makes this structure and shape occur a cause.

QUESTION EIGHTEEN: How is cool urine heated and how is hot urine cooled?

ANSWER: This is recorded in the first treatise of Galen's *al-Adwiya al-mufrada*,[21] where he says: Cool urine is frequently a reason **[56a]** for the withdrawal of [innate] heat by means of cooling the humor and collecting it (the humor) in it (the urine). Hot urine frequently becomes cool by means of dissolving the humor, which is warm.

QUESTION NINETEEN: How many conditions are there which, if they occur together, the initial cause affects the body as an illness?

ANSWER: This is recorded in Ibn Riḍwān's *al-Uṣūl*. Three. First is that the body is ready for that illness, that is, it is susceptible to that cause. Second is that the magnitude of the cause is very great or its strength is excessive, which would enable it to change the body. Third is that it (the illness) remains in contact with the body like this for sufficient time, allowing the body to change by means of it.

QUESTION TWENTY: How many occasions are there for a susceptible organ to accept [an illness]?

ANSWER: Seven. First, [depending on] the accumulation of its (the illness') superfluity in the repelling organ. Second, the strength of the repelling [organ]. Third, the weakness of the susceptible organ. Fourth, the width of the vessels. Fifth, the [degree of] porosity of the mass of the susceptible organ at the bottom, so that it [is able to] overcome the substance [of the illness] at the bottom. Seventh,[22] the narrowness of the vessels into which the susceptible organ pushes its excess.

We ask almighty God to inspire us with obedience to Him, to make us follow the path of His favor in worshipping Him, to make us gather in

[21] On the *Kitāb fī l-Adwiya al-mufrada* ["Book on Simple Drugs"], the Arabic of which has not been published, see *GAS* III, 109–10, index; Ullmann, *Medizin*, pp. 47–48.

[22] The sixth is missing.

the abode of His magnanimity, and to bestow upon us the intercession of Muḥammad, lord of the prophets, may God bless him and all his pure family and companions, by the leave of God, may he be exalted and glorified.

BIBLIOGRAPHY

This bibliography includes all those items cited in the text or notes of the present work with the exception of articles from the *EI*. In alphabetizing romanized Arabic names and titles, the definite article "al-" has been ignored, as also have differences between the transliterated forms of Arabic letters represented by the same Latin character (e.g., *d* and *ḍ*, *u* and *ū*).

Abū Shāma 'Abd al-Raḥmān ibn Ismā'īl. *Al-Dhayl 'alā l-Rawḍatayn*. Pub. under the title *Tarājim rijāl al-qarnayn al-sādis wa-l-sābi'*. Cairo: 'Izzat al-'Aṭṭār al-Ḥusaynī, 1366/1947.

'Alī ibn 'Īsā al-Kaḥḥāl. *Tadhkirat al-kaḥḥālīn*. Ed. Ghawth Muḥyī l-Dīn al-Qādirī. Hyderabad, Deccan: Dā'irat al-Ma'ārif al-'Uthmāniyya, 1964.

Anonymous. *Tuḥfat al-aḥbāb: glossaire de la matière médicale morocaine*. Ed. and trans. H.P.J. Renand and Georges S. Colin. Paris: Paul Geuthner, 1934.

Arberry, Arthur J. *The Koran Interpreted*. 2 parts in 1 vol. New York: Macmillan, 1970.

Aristophanes. *Lysistrata*. Norwalk, Connecticut: The Easton Press, 1983.

Ashtor, Eliyahu. *Histoire des prix et des salaires dans l'orient médiéval*. Paris: Centre national de la recherche scientifique, 1969.

Bauer, T. *Das Pflanzenbuch des Abū Ḥanīfa ad-Dīnawarī. Inhalt, Aufbau, Quellen*. Wiesbaden: Harrassowitz, 1988.

BEO = *Bulletin des études orientales*.

BHM = *Bulletin of the History of Medicine*.

Brockelmann, Carl. *Geschichte der arabischen Litteratur*. 2nd ed., 2 vols. Leiden: E.J. Brill, 1943–49. *Supplement*. 3 vols. Leiden: E.J. Brill, 1937–42.

BSOAS = *Bulletin of the School of Oriental and African Studies*.

Bürgel, J.C. "Secular and Religious Features of Medieval Arabic Medicine," in Charles Leslie, ed., *Asian Medical Systems: A Comparative Study* (Berkeley: University of California Press, 1976), pp. 44–62.

Burton, Richard, trans. *Supplemental Nights to the Book of the Thousand Nights and a Night*. 6 vols. Benares = Stoke Newington, London, 1886–88.

Cahen, Claude. "'Abdallaṭīf al-Baghdādī, portraitiste et historian de son temps," *BEO* 23 (1970), pp. 101–28.

Chardin, John. *Travels in Persia 1673–1677*. New York: Dover, 1988.

Conrad, Lawrence I. "Usāma ibn Munqidh and Other Witnesses to Frankish and Islamic Medicine in the Era of the Crusades," in Efraim Lev, ed., *Medicine in Jerusalem through the Ages* (Tel Aviv: Bar Elan University Press, 1998), pp. 1–26.

——. "Scholarship and Social Context: A Medical Case From the Eleventh-Century Near East," in Don Bates, ed., *Knowledge and the Scholarly Medical Traditions* (Cambridge: Cambridge University Press, 1995), pp. 84–100.

——. "The Arab-Islamic Medical Tradition," in Conrad *et al.*, *The Western Medieval Tradition: 800 BC to AD 1800* (Cambridge: Cambridge University Press, 1995), pp. 93–138.

——. "Medicine," in John Esposito, ed., *The Oxford Encyclopedia of the Modern Middle East* (Oxford: Oxford University Press, 1995), III, 85–89.

al-Dhahabī, Abū 'Abd Allāh Muḥammad ibn Aḥmad. *Tadhkirat al-ḥuffāẓ*. 3rd rev. ed. 4 vols. Hyderabad, Deccan: Dā'irat al-Ma'ārif al-'Uthmāniyya, 1375–77/1955–58.

Dietrich, Albert. *Medicinalia Arabica*. Göttingen: Vandenhoeck and Ruprecht, 1966.

——. "Islamic Sciences and the Medieval West: Pharmacology," in Khalil I. Semaan, ed., *Islam and the Medieval West* (Albany: State University of New York Press, 1980), pp. 50–63.

al-Dīnawarī, Abū Ḥanīfa Aḥmad ibn Dāwūd. *Kitāb al-Nabāt*. Vol. I, ed. Bernard Lewin, *The Book of Plants of Abū Ḥanīfa ad-Dīnawarī*. Uppsala: Lundequistska Bokhandeln, 1953; vol. II, ed. Muḥammad Hamīd Allāh. Cairo: Institut français d'archéologie orientale, 1973.

Dodge, Bayard, trans. *The Fihrist of al-Nadīm*. 2 vols. New York: Columbia University Press, 1970.

Dols, Michael W. *Medieval Islamic Medicine: Ibn Riḍwān's Treatise "On the Prevention of Bodily Ills in Egypt."* Berkeley: University of California Press, 1984.

——. *Majnūn: The Madman in Medieval Islamic Society*. Oxford: Oxford University Press, 1992.

——. "Leprosy in Medieval Arabic Medicine," *JHMAS* 34 (1979), pp. 314–33.

——. "The Leper in Medieval Islamic Society," *Speculum* 58 (1983), pp. 891–916.

——. "The Origins of the Islamic Hospital: Myth and Reality," *BHM* 61 (1987), pp. 367–90.

Dozy, R.P.A. *Supplément aux dictionnaires arabes*. 2nd ed. 2 vols. Leiden: E.J. Brill, 1927.

Dubler, César E., ed. and trans. *La ‚Materia Médica' de Dioscorides*. 6 vols. Barcelona: Tipografia Emporium, 1953–59.

Eddé, Anne-Marie. "Les médecins dans la société syrienne du VIIe/XIIIe siècle," *Annales Islamologiques* 29 (1995), pp. 91–109.

EI ^{1} = *Encyclopaedia of Islam*. 1st ed. Leiden: E.J. Brill, 1913–42.

EI ^{2} = *Encyclopaedia of Islam*. 2nd ed. Leiden: E.J. Brill, 1960–2002.

Eickelman, Dale F. "The Art of Memory: Islamic Education and Its Social Reproduction," *Comparative Studies in Society and History* 20 (1978), pp. 485–516.

Elisséeff, Nikita. *Nūr ad-Dīn: un grand prince musulman de Syrie au temps des croisades (511–569 H./1118–1174)*. 3 vols. Damascus: Institut français, 1967.

Fähndrich, Hartmut, ed. and trans. *Treatise to Ṣalāḥ al-Dīn on the Revival of the Art of Medicine*. Wiesbaden: Franz Steiner, 1983.

Fihrist al-kutub al-ʿarabiyya al-maḥfūẓa bi-l-kutubkhāna al-khidīwiyya al-miṣriyya. 7 vols. Cairo, AH 1306–1309.

GAL, see Brockelmann.

GAS, see Sezgin.

Goitein, S.D. "The Four Faces of Islam," in his *Studies in Islamic History and Institutions* (Leiden: E.J. Brill, 1968), pp. 3–53.

Gottschalk, Hans L. *Al-Malik al-Kāmil von Egypten und seine Zeit.* Wiesbaden: Otto Harrassowitz, 1958.

Gruner, O. Cameron. *A Treatise on the Canon of Medicine of Avicenna.* 1930; repr. New York: August M. Kelly, 1970.

Gunther, Robert T., trans. *The Greek Herbal of Dioscorides.* 1934; repr. New York: Hafner Publishing Co., 1959.

Haim, S. *New Persian–English Dictionary.* 2 vols. Tehran: Beroukhim, 1960.

Hava, J.G. *Al-Farā'id.* Beirut: Dār al-Mashriq, 1970.

Hinz, Walter. *Islamische Masse und Gewichte.* Leiden: E.J. Brill, 1970.

Hippocrates. *Hippocratic Writings.* Trans. Francis Adams in *Great Books of the Western World*, ed. Robert Maynard Hutchins, X. Chicago: Encyclopaedia Britannica, 1952; trans. J. Chadwick *et al.* Harmondsworth, UK: Penguin Books, 1983.

Hirschberg, J., *et al.*, trans. *Die Augenheilkunde des Ibn Sina.* Leipzig: Verlag von Veit und Comp., 1902.

——. trans. *ʿAlī ibn-ʿĪsā: Errinerungsbuch für Augenärzte.* Leipzig: Veit und Co., 1904.

Ḥunayn ibn Isḥāq. *Questions on Medicine for Scholars.* Trans. Paul Ghalioungui. Cairo: Al-Ahram Center for Scientific Translations, 1980.

Ibn Abī Uṣaybiʿa, Abū l-ʿAbbās Aḥmad ibn al-Qāsim. *ʿUyūn al-anbā' fī ṭabaqāt al-aṭibbā'.* Beirut: Dār Maktabat al-Ḥayāt, 1965.

Ibn Khallikān, Abū l-ʿAbbās Aḥmad ibn Muḥammad. *Wafayāt al-aʿyān.* Ed. Iḥsān ʿAbbās. 8 vols. Beirut: Dār al-Thaqāfa, [1968]-72.

Ibn Shaddād, ʿIzz al-Dīn Abū ʿAbd Allāh Muḥammad ibn Ibrāhīm. *Al-Aʿlāq al-khaṭīra.* Damascus section, ed. Sāmī al-Dahhān. Damascus: Institut français, 1956.

Ibn Sīnā, Abū ʿAlī al-Ḥusayn ibn ʿAbd Allāh. *Al-Qānūn fī l-ṭibb.* 3 vols. 1294/1877; repr. Baghdad: Maktabat al-Muthannā, [1970?].

——. *Ṭabīʿiyyāt al-shifā'.* Ed. Ibrāhīm Madkūr. 5 vols. to date. Cairo: al-Maṭbaʿa al-Amīriyya, 1956–proceeding.

Ibn Wāfid, ʿAbd al-Raḥmān ibn Muḥammad. *Kitāb al-Adwiya al-mufrada.* Spanish trans. and ed. Luisa Fernanda Aguirre de Cárcer. 2 vols. Madrid: Consejo Superior de Investigaciones Científicas Agencia Española de Cooperación Internacional, 1995.

Ibn Wāṣil, Jamāl al-Dīn Muḥammad ibn Sālim. *Mufarrij al-kurūb.* Ed. Jamāl al-Dīn al-Shayyāl *et al.* 5 vols. to date. Cairo: Fouad I University Press, 1953–proceeding.

Isaacs, H.D. "A Medieval Arab Medical Certificate," *Medical History* 35 (1991), pp. 250–57.

Iskandar, Albert Z. *Galen: On Examinations by Which the Best Physicians are Recognized.* Berlin: Akademie-Verlag, 1988.

Jadon, Samira. "The Physicians of Syria during the Reign of Ṣalāḥ al-Dīn 570–589 A.H./1174–1193 A.D.," *JHMAS* 25 (1970), pp. 323–40.

JHMAS = *Journal of the History of Medicine and Allied Sciences.*

Karmi, Ghada. "State Control of the Physicians in the Middle Ages: An Islamic Model," in A.W. Russell, ed., *The Town and State Physicians in Europe from the Middle Ages to the Enlightenment* (Wolfenbüttel: Herzog August Bibliothek, 1981), pp. 63–84.

Kazimirski, A. de Biberstein. *Dictionnaire Arabe–Français.* 1860; repr. Paris: G.-P. Maisonneuve, [1970?].

al-Kindī. See Levey.

de Koning, P., ed. and trans. *Trois traités d'anatomie arabes.* Leiden: E.J. Brill, 1903.

Lane, Edward William. *An Arabic–English Lexicon.* 8 vols. 1867; repr. Beirut: Librairie du Liban, 1968.

Lecker, Michael. *The Banū Sulaym: a Contribution to the Study of Early Islam.* Jerusalem: Magnes Press, 1989.

Leiser, Gary. "The Restoration of Sunnism in Egypt: Madrasas and Mudarrisūn 495–647/1101–1249." Ph.D. Dissertation, University of Pennsylvania 1976.

——. "Medical Education in Islamic Lands from the Seventh to the Fourteenth Century," *JHMAS* 38 (1983), pp. 48–75.

Leiser, Gary, and Noury Al-Khaledy. "Bilinen en eski hekimlik sınavı," *Hacettepe Üniversitesi Edebiyat Fakültesi Dergisi* 5 (1987), pp. 166–84.

Leiser, Gary, and Michael Dols. "Evliyā Chelebi's Description of Medicine in Seventeenth-Century Egypt," *Sudhoffs Archiv*, pt. 1, 71 (1987), pp. 197–216; and pt. 2, 72 (1988), pp. 49–68.

Levey, Martin, trans. *The Medical Formulary or Aqrābādhīn of al-Kindī.* Madison: University of Wisconsin Press, 1966.

——, trans. *Medieval Arabic Toxicology: The Book on Poisons of Ibn al-Waḥshīya and Its Relation to Early Indian and Greek Texts. Transactions of the American Philosophical Society*, New Series, 56.7. Philadelphia, 1966.

——, trans. *Medical Ethics of Medieval Islam with Special Reference to al-Ruhāwī's "Practical Ethics of the Physician."* Philadelphia: American Philosophical Society, 1967.

——. *Early Arabic Pharmacology.* Leiden: E.J. Brill, 1973.

——, and Noury Al-Khaledy, trans. *The Medical Formulary of al-Samarqandī.* Philadelphia: University of Pennsylvania Press, 1967.

Loebenstein, Helen. *Katalog der arabischen Handschriften der Österreichischen Nationalbibliothek.* Vienna: Hollinek in Komm., 1970.

Maimonides, Moses. *Sharḥ asmā' al-'uqqār.* Trans. and ed. Max Meyerhof in *Mémoires Présentés à l'Institut d'Égypte*, vol. 41. Cairo: Institut français d'archéologie orientale, 1940. English trans. and ed. Fred Rosner as *Moses Maimonides' Glossary of Drug Names.* Philadelphia: American Philosophical Society, 1979.

——. *Treatise on Poisons and Their Antidotes*. Trans. Suessman Muntner. Philadelphia and Montreal: Lippincott, 1966.

al-Majūsī, 'Alī ibn al-'Abbās. *Kāmil al-ṣinā'a al-ṭibbiyya* (or *al-Malakī*). 2 vols. Cairo: Būlāq, 1294/1877.

Makdisi, George. *The Rise of Colleges: Institutions of Learning in Islam and the West*. Edinburgh: Edinburgh University Press, 1981.

al-Malakī, see al-Majūsī.

McDonald, A. "Primates and Other Animals Use Wild Plants for Medicinal Purposes Researchers Discover," *The Chronicle of Higher Education*, 19 February 1992, pp. A9, A12.

Meyerhof, Max, ed. and trans. *The Book of the Ten Treatises on the Eye Ascribed to Hunain Ibn Is-Hāq*. Cairo: Government Press, 1928.

Minorsky, Vladimir, trans. *Ḥudūd al-'ālam*. London: Luzac, 1937.

al-Nu'aymī, 'Abd al-Qādir ibn Muḥammad. *Al-Dāris fī ta'rīkh al-madāris*. Ed. Ja'far al-Ḥasanī, 2 vols. Damascus: Maṭba'at al-Sharqī, 1367–70/1948–51.

al-Qānūn, see under Ibn Sīnā.

al-Rāzī, Abū Bakr Muḥammad ibn Zakariyyā. *Kitāb al-Ḥāwī fī l-ṭibb*. 23 vols. to date. Hyderabad, Deccan: Dā'irat al-Ma'ārif al-'Uthmāniyya, 1374/1955–proceeding.

——. *Kitāb al-Murshid aw al-Fuṣūl*. Ed. A.Z. Iskandar in *Majallat al-Ma'had al-Makhṭūṭāt al-'Arabiyya* 7 (1961), pp. 1–125.

Richards, D.S., ed. *Islamic Civilization 950–1150*. Oxford: Cassirer, 1973.

Riddle, John M. *Dioscorides on Pharmacy and Medicine*. Austin, Texas: University of Texas Press, 1985.

Rosenthal, Franz. "The Defense of Medicine in the Medieval Muslim World," *BHM* 43 (1969), pp. 519–32.

——. "The Physician in Medieval Muslim Society," *BHM* 52 (1978), pp. 475–91.

Sabra, A.I. "The Scientific Enterprise," in Bernard Lewis, ed., *Islam and the Arab World* (New York: Alfred Knopf, 1976), pp. 181–92.

Sadek, M.M. *The Arabic Materia Medica of Dioscorides*. Quebec: Les Editions du Sphinx, 1983.

al-Ṣafadī, Khalīl ibn Aybak. *Al-Wāfī bi-l-wafayāt*. Ed. Hellmut Ritter *et al*. 24 vols. to date. Istanbul: Staatsdruckerei, 1931–proceeding.

al-Sam'ānī, Abū Sa'd 'Abd al-Karīm ibn Muḥammad. *Kitāb al-Ansāb*. Ed. D.S. Margoliouth. Leiden: E.J. Brill, 1912.

al-Samarqandī. See Levey and Al-Khaledy.

Schacht, Joseph and Max Meyerhof. *The Medico-Philosophical Controversy Between Ibn Butlan of Baghdad and Ibn Ridwan of Cairo*. Faculty of Arts Publication No. 13, the Egyptian University. Cairo, 1937.

Sergeant, R.B. "The Cultivation of Cereals in Mediaeval Yemen," *Arabian Studies* 1 (1974), pp. 25–74.

Şeşen, Ramazan. "Eyyūbiler devrinde tip eğitimi," *İslam Tetkikleri Dergisi* 9 (1995), pp. 221–42.

Sezgin, Fuat. *Geschichte des arabischen Schrifttums*. 9 vols. Leiden: E.J. Brill, 1967–84.

Shah, Mazhar H., trans. *The General Principles of Avicenna's Canon of Medicine*. Karachi: Naveed Clinic, 1966.

Steingass, F. *Persian–English Dictionary*. 1892; repr. Beirut: Librairie du Liban, 1975.

al-Subkī, Tāj al-Dīn ʿAbd al-Wahhāb ibn ʿAlī. *Ṭabaqāt al-shāfiʿiyya al-kubrā*. Ed. Maḥmūd Muḥammad al-Ṭanāḥī and ʿAbd al-Fattāḥ Muḥammad al-Ḥilū. 10 vols. Cairo: ʿsā al-Ḥalabī, 1383–[96]/1964–[76].

Temkin, Owsei. *Galenism: The Rise and Fall of a Medical Philosophy*. Ithaca, New York: Cornell University Press, 1973.

Thakral, K.K. "Techniques for Extraction of Foreign Bodies from War Wounds in Medieval India," *Indian Journal of the History of Science* 16i (1981), pp. 11–16.

Ṭuḥfa, see Anonymous, *Ṭuḥfat al-aḥbāb*.

Ullmann, Manfred. *Die Medizin im Islam*. Leiden and Köln: E.J. Brill, 1970.

——. *Islamic Medicine*. Edinburgh: Edinburgh University Press, 1978.

Wehr, Hans. *A Dictionary of Modern Written Arabic*. Ithaca, New York: Cornell University Press, 1966.

Wensinck, A.J. *A Handbook of Early Muhammadan Tradition*. Leiden: E.J. Brill, 1960.

Wood, C.A. *Memorandum Book of a Tenth-Century Oculist*. Chicago: Northwestern University Press, 1936.

Wrangham, Richard W. and Jane Goodall. "Chimpanzee Use of Medicinal Leaves," in Paul G. Heltne and Linda A. Marquardt, eds., *Understanding Chimpanzees* (Cambridge, Massachusetts: Harvard University Press, 1989), pp. 22–37.

Yāqūt ibn ʿAbd Allāh al-Ḥamawī, Abū ʿAbd Allāh. *Muʿjam al-buldān*. Ed. F. Wüstenfeld. 6 vols. Leipzig: F.A. Brockhaus, 1866–73.

INDEX

sweet flag, 73
synochus, 81–82

tabasheer, 75
ṭabāshīr, 75 n. 341
tāfsiyā, 75 n. 332
*ṭal*ᶜ, 109 n. 19
tamar hindī, 75 n. 340
tamarind, 75
tamarisk, 61, 63, 66
al-Tamīmī, Muḥammad ibn Aḥmad, 27, 60–61, 63–65
tar, Iraqi, 63
taranjubīn, 60
tare, 67
ṭarfā', 61, 63, 66
taro, 71
teazel, 68
terebinth, mastic of, 100
thapsia, 75
theriac, 79
thorn, white, 68
thūm, 75 n. 323
thyme, 63, 73
thyme, wild, 74
toadstool, 75
tragacanth, 95
truffles, 72
tuberculosis, 56
tuffāḥ, 69 n. 154
ṭuḥlub, 72 n. 243
tumescence, 84
al-Turaythīthī, Muḥmmad, 3
turbad, 75 n. 322
turmeric, 60, 62, 70
turmus, 67 n. 106
turnips, 70, 88
turpeth, 75
ṭurūd, 61
tūt, 69 n. 153
tūtiyā, 87 n. 27
tutty, 87

ᶜ*ūd*, 70
ulcers, 84, 96, 99–103
ᶜ*ullayq*, 69 n. 148
Umayyad Mosque, 2, 4
ungues (odorati), 69
ᶜ*unnāb*, 67 n. 115
ᶜ*unṣul*, 74 n. 299
ushna, 68 n. 121
ushnān, 73 n. 254
ᶜ*usṭūkhūdūs*, 65 n. 57
ᶜ*urūq*, 74

verdigris, 102
vetch, 67
vinegar, 69, 88
violet, 69
vitriol, 87

wajj, 73 n. 266
walnut, Greek, 73
walnuts, 67, 70
ward, 68 n. 125
wars, 60 n. 7
wasakh al-kawā'ir, 70 n. 184
water lily, 69
water caltrop, 68
watermelon, 72
wax, 60–61, 104
willow, Egyptian, 61, 69
wormwood, 65, 75, 80
wushshāq, 73 n. 265

yabrūḥ, 75 n. 335
yanbūt, 74 n. 290
yarbaṭūra, 73 n. 282
yāsamīn, 70 n. 190
Yemen, 61–62

*za*ᶜ*farān*, 70
zāj, 87 n. 23
zanjabīl, 75 n. 329
zarāwand, 70 n. 185
zarnab, 73
*za*ᶜ*rūr*, 68 n. 136
zaytūn, 92 n. 10
zift, 73 n. 268
zinjār, 102 n. 21
zūfā, 61 n. 28
zurunbād, 70

Printed in the United States
By Bookmasters

كتاب

إمتحان الألباء لكافة الأطباء

تأليف

موفق الدين عبد العزيز بن عبد الجبار

بن أبي محمد السلمي الدمشقي المتوفي سنة ٦٠٤ هـ/١٢٠٨م

حققه وترجمه إلى الإنكليزية

جاري لايزِر ونوري الخالدي

طبع في مدينة ليدن

بمطبعة بريل

سنة ٢٠٠٤

بسم اللّه الرحمن الرحيم[1]

[المقدمة]

الحمد للّه الذي أمدّ بفوائد الحكم وأسبغ فواضل النعم وخلق الإنسان وعلّمه ما لم يعلم، وجعل له من الحيوان والنبات والمعادن[2] ما يحفظ الصحة بإذنه ويزيل السقم، وصلى اللّه على سيدنا محمد خاتم الرسل وعلى[3] آله وسلم.

أما بعد، فإن العلوم قد أشرقت نيّراتها، وظهرت بعد الخمول أياتها، وقويت أنفس أربابها، وعلت[4] همم طلابها، وقام سوق[5] الفضائل، وتلا ذوو المعارف في هذه الدولة الكريمة. وقل جاء الحق وزهق الباطل.

فأما علم الأديان فقد قام مجده /2a/ لا زال قائماً، وعز جانبه لا برح عزه ملازماً، تشيدت أركانه، وطاب لطالبه زمانه، كل ذلك بالنظر الأسنى من المقام الأسمى، سيد الوزراء، مالك الأعناق، الصاحب[6] بقية السلف مفتي الفريقين[7] صفي الدين عبد اللّه بن علي لا زالت الأفلاك لأمره طائعة وتيجان الأملاك في مقامه ساجدة راكعة ما بدت شمس طالعة وسحت سحب هامية هامعة، الصاحب الذي لا رادّ من البشر لما أراد. فهو بحر العلوم الذي لا يفتر تياره، وبدر المجد الذي لا تنكسف أنواره وسراج الفضل الذي لا تخبو[8] ناره، وغمام الكرم الذي لا تنقطع[9] أمطاره. قد إستولى/2b/ على أمد الكمال فلن يوصل إليه وإستعلى[10] على

درك الغاية فلم يزاحم عليه. فهو من الدهر نسيج[11] وحده، ومن الفخر واسطة عِقده فلو ناجا النظم قوافيه لقال فيه:

إذا ما راية رفعت لمجد، تلقتها يمينك واليسار
وإن ما غارة شنت لفقر، تعقبها الغني بك واليسار

جمع أشتات الفضائل وملك أعناق الأحرار بالحزم والعزم[12] ولله درّ[13] القائل:

خلقت بلا مشاكلة لشيء فأنت الفوق والثقلان دون[14] شمس الإيمان مشرقة في سماء محياه وآيات أنوارها تهدي لميت الضلال هداه ومحياه تلوح[15] في أفق الظلماء غرته كأنها ملة الإسلام في الملل. فآياته الباهرة لا يحصى عددها ولا يحصر، ولا ينسى محفوظها ولا يستر. فالقوة الإنسانية عاجزة عن إستيعاب فضائله معترفة بالتقصير عن أداء فرض مدحه ونوافله وفيه أقول:

لو شغلنا[16] بمدحك الأعمارا وطوينا الدهور والأعصارا
وإستعنا بكل فكر ورضنا في مداك الأسماع والأبصارا
وإنتحلنا الألفاظ نظماً و نثراً والمعاني وتصفحاً إعتبارا
/3a/ ثم أفضى بنا المقال إلى ما لا يناهي[17] له لعد إختصارا
أيها الصاحب المليك ومن حاز علواً وسؤدداً وفخارا
دمت في عزة ورفعة شأن وسعود مخلد[18] لن تبارا

فالمقام الصاحبي أعلاه الله أولى من عذر وأشرف من سلا[19] عن التجاوز فصفح وغفر.

وأما علم الأبدان، فالأمل فيه أدام الله أيامه نضارة[20] عوده ونجاز وعوده

وتحلية حاله، وتبليغ المعنى به من العزّ في هذه الدولة الكريمة غاية آماله ليظهر علم الأبدان في نمط إظهار علم الأديان، فهو علم يعرف به أحوال بدن الإنسان، أعماله طاعات للّه، وذلك إن اللّه سبحانه خلق لعبّاده من الأدوية بكل ناحية[21] ما تخلصهم من الأمراض. وجعل في الإنسان العقل آلة يستخرج بها منافعه وعلّمه إستخراج الأدوية بصناعة الطب. وألهم الحيوان الذي لا عقل له معرفة ما يحتاج إليه من الأدوية، فترى الحيوان يعرف الأدوية النافعة من غير تعليم من ذلك. إن الأيل[22] يجتذب الأفعى من قرارها بإستنشاقه نفسه حتى يخرجها ويبرزها إليه قسراً. فيغتذي بها وهي في ذلك تلدغ شفتيه /3b/ وهو لا يكترث. ثم إنه يبادر بعد أكله إياها إلى السراطين النهرية فيأكلها في أثر أكله الأفاعي[23] ليدفع بذلك ضرر السم من الحيات، فيقوم أكله السراطين مقام الترياق. ثم إنه يصبر على الظمأ الشديد، ويطاول العطش المفرط لعلمه أنه إن شرب الماء البارد على أثر لدغ الأفاعي هلك. فهو يأتي الماء فينظر إليه من بعد و لا يشربه خوفاً من الهلاك. وهذا إلهام من اللّه سبحانه.

ولقد رأيت في رسالة التميمي أن السقنقور إذا عض إنساناً فهو يسابقه إلى الماء أو إلى أن يبول و يتمرغ فيه. فإن سبق السقنقور إلى الماء أو بال[24] وتمرغ فيه مات المعضوض. وإن سبق المعضوض إلى أحدهما مات السقنقور. ومنها إن الذئب إذا وطئ نبت الإشقيل، خدرت قوائمه ولم يقدر على الحركة، فيأخذها[25] الثعلب ويتحصن به خوفاً من أن يأتي الذئب إلى جرائه فيأكلها. ولقد رأيت في طبيعيات الشفاء لإبن سينا[26] أن الفهد إذا أكل من الدواء المعروف بخانق النمر، عمد إلى زبل

الإنسان فأكله فيشفى وأن السلحفاة إذا أكلت الحية تأكل بعد ذلك من الصعتر الجبلي وأمثال هذه الأشياء كثيرة.

فصناعة الطب يتوصل بها إلى إجتلاب المنافع وإجتناب المضار، فيحتاج الطبيب أن يكون لطيف الحسّ، حسن الحدس /4a/ ذكي القلب، حديد الذهن، صحيح الفكر، جيد الذكر، صادق القول، ناصحاً لمن إستنصحه، كثير المطالعة، ملازماً للقراءة[27] وقد ذكر جالينوس في الميامر في باب السعفة أن الطبيب يحتاج أن تجتمع فيه أربعة أشياء: أحدها أن يكون ورعاً ذا فطنة ودين و فهم، الثاني أن يكون ذا علم و خبرة بطبائع العلل التي يتولى علاجها[28]، الثالث أن يكون ذا علم وخبرة بطبائع الأعلاء الذين يعالجهم[29]، الرابع أن يكون ذا علم وخبرة بقوى الأدوية، فهي صناعة سنية، ورتبتها عند ذوي الرتب علية.

رأيت لإبن الجوزي كتاباً في صناعة الطب يقول فيه: حكي عن شيث بن آدم عليهما السلام، أنه أظهر الطب وأنه ورثه عن آدم. قال: وحدثنا أبو سعيد أحمد بن محمد بأسناد بلغ فيه سعيد بن جبير عن إبن عباس عن النبي صلى اللّه عليه وسلم[30] أنه قال: كان سليمان بن داود عليه السلام[31]، إذا صلى رأى شجرة ثابتة بين يديه. فيسألها ما إسمك؟ فإن كانت لغرس غرست، وإن كانت لدواء كتبت. وروي عن أُسامة بن شريك قال: كنت عند النبي صلى اللّه عليه وسلم، وجاءت الأعراب فقالوا: يا رسول اللّه أنتداوى؟ قال: نعم، يا عبّاد اللّه تداووا، فإن /4b/ اللّه عزّ وجلّ، لم يصنع داء إلا وضع له شفاء غير داء واحد. قالوا: وما هو، يا رسول اللّه؟ قال: الهرم.

قال الأحنف بن قيس: أربع يسود بهن المرء، العلم والأدب والعفّة[32] والأمانة، وثلاث لا ينبغي للعاقل أن يدعهن: علم يحثه على عمل، وطب يذبّ به عن جسده، وصناعة يستعين بها على أمر معاشه.

وقد روي عن الشافعي رحمه اللّه أنه قال: العلم علمان، علم للدين وعلم للدنيا فالذي للدين هو الفقه و الذي للدنيا هو الطب وعنه رحمه اللّه[33] أنه قال: صنفان لا غناء بالناس عنهما، الأطباء لأبدانهم والفقهاء لأديانهم. وقد قيل: لا ينبغي للعاقل أن يسكن بلداً ليس فيه خمس، سلطان عادل، وقاضٍ عالم، وطبيب ماهر، وسوق قائمة، ونهر جارٍ.

وأما أهل هذه الصناعة في المقام الصاحبي أسماه اللّه، حسم مواد الضرر بمنع[34] من[35] تطاول[36] إليها وليست عنده أهلية ولا له من العلم مزية لأنها مرخاة الخطام، مطلقة الزمام، مهيلة المسالك، مركوبة الأخطار والمهالك. فالحجام المزين يداوي أمراض العين والجراح، والكحّال يداوي أمراض البدن لأنّ الباب مباح.

فرحم اللّه عبد العزيز، لقد حاز في مدة ولايته القليلة ثناء جزيلاً وذكراً جميلاً ودعا للمقام الصاحبي إذ ولاه دهراً طويلاً /5a/ وبعد، فلما كانت عادة المملوك أن يخدم الجناب العالى الصاحبي أعلاه اللّه بخدمة تدرس ولا تندرس لأنها تنقل من السطور إلى الصدور، سلك ذلك المسلك وعمل هذا المختصر يتبين به معرفة مدعي هذه الصناعة ومقدار فهمه، ويظهر به جودة عمله وعلمه. وقسمته إلى أبواب عشرة، في كل باب عشرون مسألة، لا يسع أدنى طبيب إلا أن يكون على خاطره وذكره. ولم أذكر إلا المشهور المنصوص. ثم ذكرت أجوبتها والمكان الذي

أخذت منه، ليكون حجة للسائل إذا جاوبه المسؤول بغير الجواب قيل له هذه المسألة مسطورة، ذكرها فلان في كتاب كذا وكذا، في موضع كذا وكذا[37] . وليس لي في ذلك سوى الجمع لهذه المسائل وإلتقاطها من كتب الأوائل وسميته إمتحان الألباء لكافة الأطباء والله سبحانه وتعالى[38] يوفقني بخدمة المقام الصاحبي في كل زمان ويجعلني من قوم قال الله فيهم: "يستبشرون برحمة منه ورضوان."

الباب الأول في النبض ومعرفته.

الباب الثاني في البول ودلالته.

الباب الثالث في الحميات والبحارين.

الباب الرابع في العلامات الجيدة والمخوفة /5b/.

الباب الخامس في الأدوية المفردة.

الباب السادس في المعالجات.

الباب السابع فيما يسأل عنه الكحّال.

الباب الثامن فيما يلزم الجرائحي.

الباب التاسع فيما يسأل عنه المجبّر.

الباب العاشر في مسائل من أصول هذه الصناعة.

الباب الأول في النبض وهو عشرون مسألة[1]

السؤال الأول—هل يمكن الطبيب أن يعرف من النبض إسم المعشوق وكيف ذلك؟

الجواب—هذا منقول من جزئيات القانون لإبن سينا حيث يقول[2]: العشق مرض وسواسي يكون النبض فيه[3] مختلفاً بلا نظام[4] كنبض أصحاب الهم[5] حتى أنه[6] يستدلّ من النبض على إسم[7] المحبوب[8] وطريق[9] ذلك هو[10] أن تذكر[11] أسماء كثيرة وتكون[12] اليد على النبض[13] فإذا إختلف عند ذكر شخص[14] إختلافاً عظيماً فصف[15] شكله وشخصه وكرّر عليه ذكره فإن تزايد إختلافه[16] وصار شبيهاً بالمنقطع[17] فقد[18] عرفت[19] إسم المحبوب.

السؤال الثاني—كم هي الأشياء /6a/ التي يحتاج المتدرّب في النبض إلى تعريفها؟

الجواب—خمسة[20]، هذا منقول من المقالة الخامسة من النبض الكبير لجالينوس حيث يقول: أول ما يحتاج الطبيب أن يتعرّفه[21] من النبض مقدار الإنبساط، الثاني زمان الحركة، الثالث حال القوّة التي تحرك العرق الضارب، الرابع حال صفاق العرق وقرعه، الخامس أن يعرف زمان السكون.

السؤال[22] الثالث—كم هي المزاوجات[23] الحاصلة للنبض إذا كان المغير له الحاجة

والقوّة وكيف يكون النبض؟

الجواب—أربعة، هذا منقول من المقالة التاسعة من كتاب النبض الكبير لجالينوس حيث يقول: الأول أن تكون القوّة كثيرة الضعف مع حرارة زائدة تجعل النبض صغيراً بطيئاً متواتراً جداً. الثاني، قوّة ضعيفة مع فتور الحرارة الغريزية وضعفها تجعل النبض خاملاً ويكون خموله بسبب ما يخور من القوّة ويكون من الصغر والإبطاء كالمزاوجة الأولى إلا أنه دون الغاية القصوى في التواتر. الثالث، قوّة زائدة وحرارة زائدة معاً تجعل النبض شديداً جداً، عظيماً جداً، ولا يكون سريعاً جداً. الرابع، صحة القوّة وعوز الحرارة تجعل النبض معتدلاً في العظم كثير /6b/ الإبطاء في غاية التفاوت وخاصة إذا كانت البرودة قد قويت كثيراً.

السؤال الرابع—من أين[24] يعلم أن في النبض طبيعة موسيقاوية؟

الجواب—هذا منقول من الكلّيّات لإبن سينا حيث يقول: كما أن صناعة الموسيقى تتم بتأليف النغم علي نسبة[25] في الحدة والثقل وبأدوار إيقاع مقدار الأزمنة التي تتخلل نقراتها كذلك الحال في[26] النبض فإن نسبة ازمنتها في السرعة والتواتر نسبة إيقاعية ونسبة أحوالها في القوّة والضعف[27] نسبة تأليفية[28]، وكما إن أزمنة الإيقاع ومقادير النغم قد تكون متفقة[29] وغير متفقة، كذلك الإختلافات قد تكون منتظمة[30] وغير منتظمة، وأيضاً بنسب[31] أحوال النبض في القوّة والضعف والمقدار قد تكون متفقة وقد تكون غير متفقة.

السؤال الخامس—في كم أمر تكون الإعتبارات التي يعتبر بها تشابه أجزاء نبضة أو تشابه جزء واحد من النبضة؟

الجواب—هذا منقول من الكلّيّات لإبن[32] سينا، في أمور خمسة في العظم والصغر والقوّة والضعف والسرعة والبطء والتفاوت والتواتر[33] والصلابة واللين.

السؤال السادس—/7a/ كيف يغير النوم النبض على الإمتلاء أو الخوى، وكيف يكون النبض عند اليقظة، إما طبيعية وإما بسبب يرد[34] من خارج؟

الجواب—هذا منقول من الكلّيّات لإبن سينا حيث يقول: النبض تختلف أحكامه بحسب الوقت من النوم، وبحسب حال الهضم. فالنبض[35] في أول النوم صغير ضعيف لأن الحرارة الغريزية حركتها في ذلك الوقت إلى الإنقباض والغوور لا إلى الإنبساط والظهور لأنها في ذلك الوقت تتوجه بكليتها بتحريك النفس لها إلى الباطن لهضم الغذاء وإنضاج الفضول و[36] تكون[37] أشدّ إبطاء وتفاوتاً لأن[38] الحرارة الغريزية[39] وإن حدث فيها تزيد بحسب الإحتقان[40]، فقد عدمت التزيد الذي كان[41] لها في حال اليقظة بحسب الحركة المسخنة. فإذا إستمرئ الطعام في النوم عاد النبض فقوي لتزيد القوّة بالغذاء وإنصراف ما كان إتجه إلى الغور لتدبير الغذاء[42] فيعظم النبض. فإذا تمادى[43] النوم عاد النبض ضعيفاً لإحتقان الحرارة الغريزية وإنضغاط القوّة تحت الفضول التي من حقها أن تستفرغ بأنواع الإستفراغ الذي يكون باليقظة التي منها الرياضات والإستفراغات[44]. فإذا صادف النوم من أول الوقت خلاء فيدوم الصغر والبطء والتفاوت في النبض. فإذا إستيقظ[45] بطبعه مال النبض إلى العظم والسرعة[46] متدرجاً[47] وإن[48] /7b/ إستيقظ[49] بسبب مفاجئ جعل النبض عظيماً مختلفاً[50] إلى الإرتعاش، ثم يعاود إلى الإعتدال سريعاً[51].

السؤال السابع—ما سبب النبض المنشاري؟

الجواب—هذا منقول من الكلّيّات لإبن سينا حيث يقول: سبب النبض المنشاري إختلاف المصبوب في جرم العرق في عنفه وفجاجته ونضجه. وإختلاف أحوال العرق في صلابته ولينه وورم في الأعضاء العصبانية. إبن التلميذ يقول على ذلك: السبب في منشارية النبض لصاحب ذات الجنب ونحوها غير ما ذكره وهو إرتفاع أجزاء للحاجة و إنخفاض أجزاء للألم والإنفعال من موجبه هذا في الشرايين التي تنبض في نفس الورم ثم تتعدى تلك الحركات المختلفة إلى سائر الشرايين لأن فاعل الإنبساط والمنفعل بالأذى واحد وهو القوّة الحيوانية.

السؤال الثامن—لم كان نبض أصحاب الإستسقاء المائي مائلاً[52] إلى الصلابة؟

الجواب—هذا منقول من النبض الكبير لجالينوس حيث يقول: نبض أصحاب الإستسقاء المائي مائل إلى الصلابة من قبل أنه تجتمع فيه رطوبة كثيرة فيما يحويه البطن قد ينال العروق الضوارب من تلك الرطوبة آفة على طريق المشاركة فبسبب تمدد العرق يجعله مائلاً إلى الصلابة /8a/ وبسبب ما ينال القوة من الآفة والمضرة وبسبب برد العرق يصير النبض أصغر وبمقدار[53] ما يصير عليه من الصغر يكون أشد تواتراً لا سيّما متى[54] كان مع هذه العلة حمى.

السؤال التاسع—ما نبض أصحاب اليرقان من غير حمى ولم ذلك؟

الجواب—هذا منقول من المقالة الثالثة عشر من النبض الكبير لجالينوس حيث يقول: نبض أصحاب اليرقان من غير حمى صغير صلب شديد التواتر وليس بضعيف ولا سريع. وإما لم كان فهو يقول: لأن من شأن المرة الصفراء أن تجفف

بمنزلة ما يجفف الماء المالح وبهذا السبب[55] يجعل صفاق العرق أجف وأصلب وإما الصغر فلأن الآلة الصلبة لا تستطيع أن تنبسط إنبساطاً تاماً ولذلك صار مقدار تواتره بحسب مقدار زيادته في الصغر وليس هو بضعيف لأن القوّة ليست بضعيفة ولا سريعة[56] لأنه خال من الحمى فمتى كان مع حمى كان النبض سريعاً من قبل الحاجة.

السؤال العاشر—ما هو النبض الحسن الوزن وما هو مجانب الوزن وما هو مخالف الوزن وما هو خارج الوزن؟

الجواب—هذا منقول من المقالة الأولى من النبض الكبير لجاليوس حيث يقول: إن في كل سن من الأسنان للعرق وزناً ما طبيعياً، فإن لزمه الوزن /8b/ سمي حسن الوزن وإن غادره قليلاً وكان الغادر للوزن الطبيعي موافقاً لوزن يكون في سن قريب من سن صاحبه سمي مجانب الوزن[57]، وإن لم يكن[58] موافقا[59] لسن قريب من سن صاحبه ثم كان موافقاً لوزن يكون في سن من الأسنان أي سن كان، قيل له مخالف الوزن وإن لم يوافق النبض نبض واحد من الأسنان قيل له خارج الوزن.

السؤال الحادي عشر—ما تقول في النبض الحسن الوزن و السيئ الوزن والمستوي والمختلف والمنتظم وغير المنتظم في كم جنس من أجناس النبض يوجد؟

الجواب—في أربعة أجناس، هذا منقول من الملكي في المقالة السابعة حيث يقول: إن النبض الحسن الوزن والسيئ الوزن والمستوي والمختلف والمنتظم وغير المنتظم لا يوجد[60] إلا في أربعة اجناس وهي الجنس الذي من كمية الإنبساط

والجنس[61] الذي من كيفية[62] الحركة والجنس الذي من مقدار القوّة والجنس الذي من وقت السكون لأن الإختلاف لا يعم سوى هذه الأربعة الأجناس.

السؤال الثاني عشر—هل بين النبض المستوي والمختلف معتدل مثل العظيم والصغير أو السريع والبطئ؟

الجواب—ليس بينهما معتدل. هذا منقول من المقالة السابعة من الجزء العلمي[63] من الملكي حيث يقول: النبض /9a/ المختلف والمستوي ليس بينهما متوسط لأن النبض المستوي هو الطبيعي الصحي والمختلف خارج عن الطبع ولا يكون إلا عن مرض والمتوسط بينهما ليس بمستوٍ.

السؤال الثالث عشر—في أي الأبدان يكون النبض أعظم، أ في الأبدان القضيفة قضفاً[64] طبيعياً أم في الأبدان العبلة ولم ذلك؟

الجواب—هذا منقول من الملكي حيث يقول: في الأبدان القضيفة[65] يكون النبض أعظم من الأبدان العبلة[66] الكثيرة اللحم وأقوى. والنبض في الأبدان العبلة أصغر وأضعف لأن الشريان في الأبدان العبلة[67] يستره ويثقله كثرة اللحم إلا أن النبض في الأبدان العبلة أشد تواتراً وذلك لضعف القوّة عن تعظيم الشريان تستعمل التواتر ليقوم لها مقام العظم.

السؤال الرابع عشر—كيف يكون نبض الحامل ولم ذلك[68] ؟

الجواب—هذا منقول من الملكي[69]، يكون نبض الحامل عظيماً شديد السرعة والتواتر لأن الحرارة في أبدان الحامل[70] قوّية بسبب ما ينضاف إلى مزاجهم من حرارة الجنين لما يتأدى من حرارته إلى شرايين المرأة لإتصال شرايين الجنين التي في المشيمة

بشرايينها إلا أنها في الشهر السادس يصير نبضها ضعيفاً بطيئاً.

السؤال الخامس عشر—ما هو النبض الخاص بكل واحد من أصناف /9b/ الإستسقاء؟

الجواب—هذا منقول من القانون لإبن سينا حيث يقول: أما الزقي فيكون النبض فيه[71] صغيراً متواتراً مائلاً إلي الصلابة مع شئ من التمدد لتمدد الحجب وربما مال في آخره إلى اللين لكثرة الرطوبة. وأما اللحمي فيكون النبض فيه[72] موجياً عريضاً ليناً [73]. وأما الطبلي [74] فيكون النبض فيه طويلاً ليس بضعيف[75].

السؤال السادس عشر—كيف يكون نبض أصحاب الهم؟

الجواب—هذا منقول من الملكي، صغير ضعيف متفاوت، فإن طال حتى ينهك القوّة فإن النبض يصير دودياً، ثم يصير نملياً عند ما تنحل القوّة وتسقط.

السؤال السابع عشر—كيف يكون نبض أصحاب الخناق وما علامات إنتقال مادته إلى ذات الرئة أو إلى ناحية القلب من جهة النبض؟

الجواب—هذا منقول من القانون لإبن سينا، أما نبض أصحاب الخناق في أوله فمتواتر مختلف ثم يصير صغيراً متفاوتاً، فإن صار النبض موجياً عظيماً وحدث سعال فهو[76] ينتقل إلى ذات الرئة، فإن[77] ضعف النبض جداً وصغر وتفاوت وحدث[78] خفقان وإنحلت الغريزية وحدث غشي، فالمادة منصبة إلى ناحية القلب.

السؤال الثامن عشر—اللذة كيف تجعل النبض؟

الجواب—/10a/ هذا منقول من المقالة الثانية عشر من النبض الكبير لجالينوس حيث يقول: اللذة تجعل النبض عظيماً متفاوتاً بطيئاً.

السؤال التاسع عشر—أيما أدل على الخوف النبض الصلب غاية الصلابة أو اللين غاية اللين؟

الجواب—كلاهما سواء هذا منقول من المقالة الرابعة عشر من النبض الكبير لجالينوس حيث يقول: وأما النبض الصلب غاية الصلابة فإنه مخوف غير مأمون على مثال اللين غاية اللين، لأن غاية الصلابة تكون إما بسبب جسا أو ورم عظيم في بعض الأحشاء، وإما بسبب جمود يحدث عن برد، وإما بسبب يبس يحدث عن حمى محرقة، وإما بسبب تشنج قوي شديد. واللين غاية اللين يكون بسبب رطوبة مفرطة جداً.

السؤال العشرون—كيف يكون النبض في الورم إذا إستحال إلى المدة؟

الجواب—هذا منقول من المقالة الثانية عشر من النبض الكبير لجالينوس حيث يقول: يكون النبض مختلفاً عديم النظام بسبب ما ينال الآلة من الآفة وبسبب ضعف القوّة ومقاومة الطبيعة للمرض ومجاهدتها.

الباب الثاني في البول وهو عشرون مسألة

/10b/ **السؤال الأول**—البول الأبيض الرقيق إذا ظهر في اليوم الرابع من المرض وتبعه علامات رديئة بماذا تحكم؟

الجواب—هذا منقول من الملكي حيث يقول: ومتى ظهر هذا البول مع أعراض رديئة في اليوم الرابع[1] فإن المريض يموت قبل السابع.

السؤال الثاني—البول الأصفر الرقيق على ماذا يدل؟

الجواب—هذا منقول من الملكي حيث يقول: يدل[2] على أن الطبيعة لم يمكنها إنضاج المادة جيداً لضعفها، وإنها قد أخذت في إنضاجها وإبتدأت باللون فغيرته إلى الصفرة. وذلك لأن الطبيعة تبتدئ أولاً بإنضاج اللون لأنه أسهل عليها ثم تأخذ بعد ذلك في إنضاج القوام.

السؤال الثالث—البول الأبيض الغليظ إذا ظهر في يوم بحران وخاصة[3] في الرابع على ماذا يدل؟

الجواب—هذا منقول من كتاب البول للإسرائيلي حيث يقول: يدل على الخلاص من أوجاع المفاصل والأورام العارضة في أصول الآذان. فإن كان ظهوره بعد البحران دل على معاودة من[4] المرض والله أعلم[5].

السؤال الرابع—البول الغليظ، إذا دام على حاله ولم يتغير زماناً على

ماذا يدل؟

الجواب—/11a/منقول من كتاب البول للإسرائيلي حيث يقول: هذا يدل على ورم يحدث فيما دون الشراسيف فإن تبعه دلائل محمودة، دل على سلامته وإلا دل على خوف.

السؤال الخامس—البول الأحمر اللطيف إذا كانت[6] له رائحة حريفة وثقل أسود كدر فيه شبيه بالشعر، ما دلالته؟

الجواب—منقول من كتاب الإسرائيلي في البول حيث يقول: هذا ردئ وهو دال على خوف.

السؤال السادس—البول الغليظ الذي لا يصفو إذا كان يصاحبه صمم ووجع في الرأس وإمتداد في الشراسيف، ما دلالته؟

الجواب—منقول من كتاب الإسرائيلي حيث يقول: هذا يدل على يرقان ردئ يحدث قبل السابع. فإن صار لطيفاً فيه تعليق كمد اللون وسائر العلامات متشابهة دل على نكسة وفساد ذهن، لاسيّما لمن يكثر من[7] الطعام.

السؤال السابع—البول الأحمر الصرف إذا كان قليلاً ويصاحبه إستسقاء، ما دلالته؟

الجواب—منقول من كتاب الإسرائيلي حيث يقول: هذا يدل على موت قريب.

السؤال الثامن—البول إذا كان على لون الدم وكان صاحبه يتقيأ شبيهاً بالزنجار /11b/ مع خشونة اللسان، ما دلالته؟

الجواب—منقول من كتاب الإسرائيلي حيث يقول: هذا يدل على شر وموت وحي.

السؤال التاسع—البول الأشقر، إذا كان له زبد كزبد الشراب، ما دلالته؟

الجواب—يدل على إختلاط عقل.

السؤال العاشر—البول الأسود متى كان رقيقاً من أول المرض، على ماذا يدل؟

الجواب—منقول من الملكي حيث يقول: يدل على الهلاك لا محالة.

السؤال الحادي عشر—كم هي أصناف الثقل الراسب؟

الجواب—منقول من الملكي حيث يقول: إنها ثلاثة، أحدها الغمامة وهو ما يتميز في أعلا القارورة، الثاني التعليق[8] وهو ما يتميز في وسطها، الثالث الرسوب[9] وهو ما يتميز في أسفلها.

السؤال الثاني عشر—البول الأخضر الدائم الخضرة إذا كان مع حمى لهبة أو لينة، ما دلالته؟

الجواب—منقول عن الإسرائيلي: إن كان مع حمى لهبة، دل على إختلاط، وإن كان مع حمى لينة وكان أكثر من مقدار ما يشرب من الماء، دل على ذوبان البدن.

السؤال الثالث عشر—/12a/ البول الأسود اللطيف مع الحمى اللهبة، إذا كان له ثقل أسود عوام لا يستقر وبصاحبه سهر وصمم، ما دلالته؟

الجواب—منقول عن الإسرائيلي: يدل على طول المرض، وإن إنحلاله

يكون بإنبعاث دم[10].

السؤال الرابع عشر—البول الأسود، إذا كان له ثقل محبب مشتر شبيه بالنقط مع نفخة في الشراسيف ووجعها، ما دلالته؟

الجواب—منقول عن الإسرائيلي حيث يقول: هذا يدل على موت.

السؤال الخامس عشر—البول الرقيق الأسود، إذا إستحال إلى الشقرة والغلظ ولم يصحب ذلك رائحة[11]، على ماذا يدل؟

الجواب—منقول من الجزئيات[12] لإبن سينا حيث يقول: هذا يدل على علة في الكبد وخصوصاً على يرقان لأن هذه الإستحالة التي إلى الغلظ عن الرقة[13] إلى الشقرة عن[14] السواد تدل[15] على نقصان حرارة ووقوع هضم[16]، وذلك مما يصحبه أو يعقبه الخف، فإن لم يكن كذلك، دل على مادة قد لحجت في الكبد ليست تستنقى، وقد أحدثت سواداً[17] فإن كانت حارة فكأنك بها قد أحدثت ورماً.

السؤال السادس عشر—/12b/ البول الغليظ الذي لا يصفو، ما دلالته؟

الجواب—منقول عن الإسرائيلي حيث يقول: هذا يدل على ريح نافخة غليظة قد خالطت الثقل وأثارته، فلذلك يدل على الصداع الحاضر أو سيحدث.

السؤال السابع عشر—البول الأحمر جداً، إذا إستحال في الحميات الإعيائية إلى الغلظ، ثم ظهر ثقل كبير لا يرسب وكان بصاحبه صداع، على ماذا يدل؟

الجواب—منقول من جزئيات القانون لإبن[18] سينا حيث يقول: هذا يدل على طول من المرض لأن المادة عاصية ولذلك[19] لم تغلظ أولاً، فلما غلظت لم ترسب

بسرعة، لكن بحرانه يكون بعرق لأن المادة مائلة إلى العروق، ومثل هذا البول يشبه اليرقان ويفارقه بأنه لا يصبغ الثوب.

السؤال الثامن عشر—البول الأحمر القاني إذا كان مع فرغ حسن، ما دلالته؟

الجواب—منقول عن الإسرائيلي حيث يقول: يدل على زوال الحمى بعد السابع.

السؤال التاسع عشر—إذا كان البول له رائحة حامضة وكانت العلة حارة، على ماذا يدل؟

الجواب—منقول من الكلّيّات حيث يقول: هذا يدل /13a/ على الموت لأنه يدل على موت[20] الحرارة الغريزية وإستيلاء برد في الطبع مع حر غريب.

السؤال العشرون—كم هي أنواع الرسوب الغير الطبيعي؟

الجواب—منقول من الكلّيّات، وهي ثمانية عشر: خراطي، و[21] نخالي، و[22] كرسني، و[23] دشيشي[24] ، و[25] شبيه بالزرنيخ الأحمر، والمشبع الصفرة، و[26] لحمي، ومخاطي، ودسمي، ومدي، وشبيه بقطع الخمير، ودموي[27]، و[28] علقي، وشعري، ورملي، و[29] حصوي، ورمادي، والله أعلم بالصواب[30].

الباب الثالث في الحميات والبحارين وهو عشرون مسألة

السؤال الأول—كم هي أصناف حمي يوم التي قسمها إبن سينا؟

الجواب—ثلاثة وعشرون، هذا منقول من الكتاب الرابع من القانون حمى غمية[1]، وهمية، وفكرية، وغضبية، وسهرية، ونومية وراحية[2]، وفرحية، وفزعية، وتعبية، وإستفراغية، ووجعية[3]، وغشية[4]، وجوعية، وعطشية، وسددية، وتخمية[5]، وورمية، وقشفية، وحرية، /13b/ وإستحصافية من البرد، وإستحصافية من ماء الشب[6]، وشربية، وغذائية[7].

السؤال الثاني—كم هي علامات حمى الغب؟

الجواب—عددها تسعة عشر، منقول من المقالة الثانية من كتاب البحران لجالينوس حيث يقول: أحدها أن يكون معها نافض[8] قوي، الثاني أن يحس كأن لحمه يغرز بالإبر، الثالث أن يكون النبض في أوائل نوائبها[9] صغيراً بطيئاً متفاوتاً إلا أن إبطاءه[10] وتفاوته ناقص عن الإبطاء والتفاوت الذين يكونان في حمى الربع نقصاناً[11] كبيراً ووقت تزيدها تكون السرعة مستوية، الرابع إن العطش والإلتهاب لا يلبث إلا حتى ينتهي منتهاها، الخامس أن تكون الحرارة منتشرة في البدن كله بالسواء، السادس أنه إذا وضعت يدك على البدن لقيتك الحرارة الكثيرة كأنها ترتفع مع بخار ثم أنها لا تلبث أن تخور[12] وتقهرها[13] يدك، السابع أن يكون عند

شرب الماء البارد يرتفع من بدنه[14] بخار حار يتقدم الجلد ينزز[15] بعرق، الثامن يتقيأ[16] مراراً أصفر، التاسع وربما إختلف مراراً وبال /14a/ بولاً يغلب فيه المرار، العاشر أن يبتدي فيه عرق بخاري حاد كالعرق الذي يعرقه الإنسان في الحمام، الحادي عشر أن يكون النبض كنبض الصحيح في حال الرياضة سريعاً عظيماً قوياً متواتراً، الثاني[17] عشر أنه ليس يتجاوز نوبة الحمى إثنا عشر ساعة وهي أطول ما يمكن، الثالث عشر إن البول يصير إلى الصفرة المشعة[18] والحمرة الناصعة معتدل الثخن وقد يحدث فيه غمامة بيضاً طافية في أعلاه أو متغلغة بوسطه، الرابع عشر أنها لا تتجاوز الدور السابع، الخامس عشر أن يكون الزمان حاراً يابساً، السادس عشر أن يكون شاباً، السابع عشر أن يكون الغالب على الطبع المرار، الثامن عشر أن يكون صاحبه يستعمل السهر والهم[19] والتعب والإقلال من الطعام، التاسع عشر أن يكون الوقت الحاضر قد غلب على الناس فيه حمى غب.

السؤال الثالث—كم هي[20] علامات حمى الربع؟

الجواب—تسع، هذا منقول من المقالة الثانية من كتاب البحران لجالينوس حيث يقول: أحدها ليس /14b/ يبتدي في أول الأمر بنافض قوي بل يحس بالبرد أكثر وهو أشبه شئ بالبرد الذي يعرض للإنسان في الشتاء عند شدة برد الهواء[21] وكان شيئاً برده ويرضّه حتى يصل إلى العظام[22]، الثاني أن يكون النبض في أوائل نوائبها صغيراً بطيئاً ضعيفاً تفاوتاً ويخيل إليك في نوائب الربع أن العرق موثوق مسدود كأنه يجذب إلى داخل ويمنع من أن يرتفع، الثالث ويكون بكثر في الخريف فإن كان الخريف مختلف المزاج قوي ظنك بأن الحمى ربعاً،الرابع أن ينظر في البلد

هل هو معين في توليدها، الخامس أن ينظر في طبيعة المريض[23] هل هي مائلة إلى السوداء[24]، السادس أن ينظر ما تقدم من تدبيره هل هو مولد للسوداء، السابع أن ينظر إن كانت عرضت لكثير من الناس، الثامن أن ينظر في البول فأنه يكون أبيض رقيقاً مائياً[25]، التاسع أن ينظر هل بالمريض طحال غليظ أو هل كانت عرضت له حمى مخلطة وقال جالينوس في المكان بعينه: ومن لم يقدر على الفرق بين حمى الربع وبين الغب منذ أول يوم، فليس من الطب في شئ.

السؤال الرابع—/15a/ كم هي علامات الحمى النائبة في كل يوم؟

الجواب—إثنا[26] عشر و هو منقول من المقالة الثانية من كتاب البحران لجالينوس حيث يقول: الأول أنها تبتدي بنافض منذ أول يوم، الثاني وأنها إذا تمادت بها الأيام يعرض فيها في أول النوائب برد ظاهر، الثالث ويوجد في النبض إختلاف ويفسد نظامه في أول النوائب وليس يوجد فيه مما[27] يوجد في الغب من السرعة والعظم والقوّة، الرابع وليس يحس فيها بتلهب شديد ولا يتنفس تنفساً عظيماً، الخامس وأن[28] يكون العطش أقل منه في سائر الحميات، السادس وأن[29] يكون البول في أول يوم منها على مثال ما يكون في أول الربع ولا يكاد المريض يعرق فيها في الأيام الأول، السابع وأن تكون طبيعة البدن رطبة ولذلك أكثر ما يعرض للصبيان، الثامن وأن تألم المعدة والكبد، التاسع وأن يتقدمها تخم[30]، العاشر وأن ينتفخ ما دون الشراسيف، الحادي عشر وأن يكون لون المريض بين الصفرة والبياض، الثاني عشر مما يعين على حدوثها المنشأ[31] والبلد.

السؤال الخامس—/15b/ كم هي العلامات الخاصية بحمى يوم؟

الجواب—ثمانية، منقول من كتاب الحميات لجالينوس، الأول ظهور النضج في البول في أول يوم، الثاني وإن يكون النبض قد تزيد[32] عظماً وسرعة تزيد إذا قدر ويكون مع ذلك إلى التواتر، الثالث أن يكون إنقباض العرق لا يزيد سرعة بتة[33] فإن يزيد[34] في بعض الحالات كان يزيده[35] يسيراً جداً وخروجه عن الحال[36] الطبيعية يسيراً، الرابع طيب الحرارة و لذاذتها، الخامس إستواء النبض، السادس تزيد[37] الحمى من غير تضاغط[38] في الحرارة و لا في النبض، السابع إنحطاط الحمى إذا كان مع عرق أو نداوة أو مع بخار رطب يتحلل من البدن ثم أتبع ذلك إقلاع تام من الحمى، الثامن وأن يكون سببها بادياً وظاهراً[39].

السؤال السادس—كم هي العلاقات الخاصة بحمى العفونة؟

الجواب—سبعة، هذا منقول من كتاب الحميات لجالينوس، أحدها أن[40] لا يتقدم هذه الحمى شئ من الأسباب الظاهرة التي تعرف بالبادية، الثاني وأن يكون في إبتدائها نافض من غير أن يكون /16a/ إصاب البدن قبل حدوثها حر شمس شديد ولا برد شديد[41]، الثالث إختلاف النبض، الرابع إختلاف الحرارة، الخامس أن يكون كيفية الحرارة غير لذيذة ولا هادية بمنزلة حمى يوم لكنها بالدخانية أشبه حمى تؤذى[42] وتقرص اللامس إلا أنها[43] في إبتداء نوبة الحمى من قبل أن الحرارة في هذا الوقت مغمورة[44] والفصول التي تعمل فيها الحرارة باطنة فلا يدرك[45] أول ما يلمس البدن فإذا طال لبث الكف على البدن إرتفعت الحرارة من العمق، السادس[46] أن لا يظهر في البول للنضج أثر، السابع وأن يظهر في وقت نوبة الحمى شيئاً من الأعراض التي تظهر في الحمى المحرقة أو من أعراض الحمى التي

يجد صاحبها البرد والحر معاً أو من أعراض الحمى التي تكون في باطن البدن حرارة شديدة وظاهره بارداً ومن أعراض شطر الغب أو من أعراض اللثقة.

السؤال السابع—لم صارت الحمى التي من عفونة الصفراء تأخذ يوماً وتترك[47] يوماً والبلغمية نائبة في كل يوم والربع تركها ضعف مدة أخذها؟

الجواب—أماالمتولدة من عفن الصفراء، فقد إجتمع فيها الحر واليبس والحرارة من شأنها دوام الحركة /16b/ وإنبساط الأجزاء[48] وهي أقوى الفاعلين[49] واليبوسة هي[50] أقوى المنفعلين[51] ومن شأنها جمع الأجزاء[52] وتقبيضها والمنع مما يوجب الحرارة فلمنع اليبوسة من دوام فعل الحرارة ما إنقطع دوام ذلك فأخذت[53] يوماً وتركت يوماً وأما النائبة[54] في كل يوم فقد إجتمع فيها[55] البرد والرطوبة والبرد من شأنه الجمع[56] والتقبيض والرطوبة من شأنها البسط والتفريق وهي عند العفونة تكون[57] القاهرة ولذلك ما يطول نوبة هذه الحمى[58] وأن يكون تركها في كل يوم ست ساعات وهو ربع يوم و ربما نقصت عن هذه وزادت وأما الربع فهي متولدة من المرة السوداء وقد إجتمع فيها البرد واليبس فالبرد أضعف الفاعلين[59] وأقلهما حركة واليبس هو[60] أقوى المتفعلين[61] ولإشتراك البرد واليبس في الجمع والتقبيض[62] وفي السكون وقلة الحركة ما تأخرت نوبة هذه العلة وتأخر دورها حتى صار تركها ضعف مدة أخذها.

السؤال الثامن—كم هي الأنحاء التي يتغير إليها المريض في البحران؟

الجواب—ستة، منقول من المقالة الثالثة من البحران لجالينوس حيث يقول: وتغير المريض[63] يكون على ستة أنحاء إما أن ينتقل دفعه[64] /17a/ إلى الصحة

ويسمى بحراناً مطلقاً وإما أن يقتل ويسمى بحراناً ردياً وإما أن ينتقل إلى الصحة[65] قليلاً قليلاً أعني[66] أن ينتقص المرض شيئاً بعد شئ ويقال له بروء وإما أن يقتل قليلاً قليلاً أعني أن تنحل قوّة المريض ويسمى بحراناً ناقصاً وإما أن يجتمع فيه الأمران ويؤول إلى الصحة وإما أن يجتمع فيه الأمران ويؤول إلى الموت.

السؤال التاسع—كم هي العلامات الدالة على جودة[67] البحران[68]؟

الجواب—خمسة، هذا منقول من المقالة الثالثة[69] من كتاب البحران له[70] الأول النضج ويقول: ما رأيت أحداً مات ممن أتاه البحران بعد النضج، الثاني أن يكون البحران في يوم من أيامه قد سبق وأنذر[71] به يوم إنذار مواصل له في قوّته، الثالث طبيعة المرض وأعني بطبيعة أن تكون الحمى غباً أو نائبة أو محرقة أو ذات جنب أو ذات رئة، الرابع سحنة أعني بالسحنة أن يكون سليماً سهلاً أو رديئاً خبيثاً[72]، الخامس أن يكون البحران مشاكلاً لطبيعة المرض.

السؤال العاشر—كيف يعرف البحران قبل حضوره؟

الجواب—منقول من المقالة الثالثة من البحران لجالينوس[73] ينظر إلي طبيعة المرض هل هو متولد من صفراء أو بلغم أو سوداء أو مختلط ثم /17b/ أنظر في أدوار النوائب[74] إذا كانت سريعة الحركة أو تنوب[75] غباً دلت على أن البحران يأتي[76] بسرعة وإذا كانت تبطئ[77] في حركتها وتبتدي[78] في وقت واحد وتنوب كل يوم دلت على أن البحران لا يأتي إلا بعد طول ثم ينظر في النضج فإنه من أقوى العلامات وينبغي[79] أن يتفقد[80] من أمر النضج التغير[81] فإن التغير إذا حدث في يوم إنذار[82] دل على أن خروج[83] المريض من علته يكون في يوم[84] البحران الذي

يتصل بذلك اليوم من أيام الإنذار.

السؤال الحادي عشر—كم هي العلامات التي تدل على البحران؟

الجواب—خمسة، هذا منقول من المقالة الأولى من كتاب أيام البحران لجالينوس حيث يقول: أولها[85] وأقواها[86] إنذار الذي قبله، الثاني قياس نوائب الحمى، الثالث طبائع الأيام، الرابع عدد أوقات البحران، الخامس زمان البحران.

السؤال الثاني عشر—في أي الأيام يكون البحران القوي؟

الجواب—هذا[87] منقول من أيام البحران لجالينوس حيث يقول: البحران القوي السابع والرابع[88] عشر والتاسع والحادي عشر والعشرون ومن /18a/ بعدها الرابع وبعده الثالث والثامن عشر.

السؤال الثالث عشر—أي الأيام التي يكون[89] فيها البحران رديئاً والتي ليست من أيام البحران؟

الجواب—منقول من كتاب أيام البحران لجالينوس، السادس وأما الثاني عشر والسادس عشر فليسا من أيام البحران وكذلك التاسع.

السؤال الرابع عشر—ما تقول في الأيام التي بعد العشرين؟

الجواب—منقول من كتاب أيام البحران لجالينوس حيث يقول: أما الحادي والعشرون فيوم بحران والعشرون منه والسابع والعشرون أيضاً فإني رأيت البحران يكون فيه أكثر ما يكون في الثامن والعشرون[90] واليوم الثلاثون[91] صالح القوّة ويوم الأربعين أقوى منه واليوم[92] الرابع والعشرون والواحد والثلاثون فالبحران فيهما على أفضل ما يكون وأقل من هذا كثيراً اليوم السابع والثلاثون

حتى إنه بين الأيام التي لا يكون فيها بحران وبين[93] الأيام الباحورية وأما بقية الأيام الآخر التي بين العشرين والأربعين فليس يكون فيها بحران.

السؤال الخامس عشر—ما هي الأيام التي فيها بين العشرين والأربعين /18b/ ولا يكون فيها بحران؟

الجواب—الثاني عشر والثاني والعشرون[94] والخامس والعشرون والسادس والعشرون والتاسع والعشرون والثلاثون والثاني والثلاثون والخامس والثلاثون والسادس والثلاثون والثامن والثلاثون[95] والتاسع والثلاثون.

السؤال السادس عشر—ما تقول في الأيام التي بعد الأربعين؟

الجواب—قال جالينوس كلها ضعيفة الحركة و إنقضاء[96] المرض فيها يكون إما بالنضج وإما بالخراجات[97] وأكثر ما يكون بالإستفراغ وقد يكون في هذه الأيام بحران بالإستفراغ لكن ذلك يكون مرة في الندرة ورأيت بقراط يستحف[98] بجميع الأيام التي بعد الأربعين خلا الستين[99] والثمانين والمائة والعشرين[100] ثم يقول جالينوس إن من الأمراض ما يكون بحرانه في سبعة أشهر ومنها ما يكون[101] في سبع سنين.

السؤال السابع عشر—بماذا يكون بحران الورم الكائن في محدب الكبد؟

الجواب—منقول من كتاب البحران لجالينوس، بأحد ثلاثة أشياء إما برعاف /19a/ من الجانب الأيمن وإما بعرق محمود وإما ببول محمود وربما كان بإثنين منهما أو بجميعها.

السؤال الثامن عشر—بماذا يكون بحران الورم الكائن في مقعر الكبد؟

الجواب—منقول من كتاب البحران لجالينوس حيث يقول: بأحد ثلاثة أشياء إما بإختلاف مرار وإما بعرق وإما بقيء.

السؤال التاسع عشر—ما هو البحران المشاكل للغب؟

الجواب—إما في مرار وإما إختلاف أو عرق كثير في البدن كله.

السؤال العشرون[102]—ما هو البحران المشاكل في النائبية؟

الجواب—إستفراغ بلغم كثير ويجري عرق كثير من البدن كله.

الباب الرابع في العلامات الجيدة والمخوفة هو عشرون مسألة[1]

السؤال الأول—إذا كان بإنسان حمى مع سعال يابس وأنقصت[2] الحمى وبقي السعال، بماذا ينذر ولم ذلك؟

الجواب—منقول من المقالة العاشرة من الملكي حيث يقول: هذا ينذر بخراجات[3] تحدث[4] في المفاصل وذلك لأن بقاء السعال يدل على بقية[5] من المادة الفاعلة /19b/ للمرض[6] لم ينضج[7] وبحران هذه المادة أكثر ما[8] يكون بخراج.

السؤال الثاني—إذا كان بياض العين أحمر وعروقها كمدة أو سود، على ماذا يدل ولم ذلك؟

الجواب—هذا منقول من المقالة العاشرة من الملكي حيث يقول: هذا يدل على الهلاك لا محالة وذلك إن إحمرار العين[9] إذا لم يكن عن رمد[10] فإنه يدل على إمتلاء الدماغ وأغشيته بمواد دموية وكمودة عروق العين وسوادها يدل على برودة العين وهذا دليل خاص على الهلاك.

السؤال الثالث—إذا كان بياض العين في وقت النوم ظاهراً ولم يكن ذلك عن عادة صحية ولايعقب إستفراغ، على ماذا يدل؟

الجواب—هذا يدل على الهلاك[11] لأنه يدل على ضعف الدماغ.

السؤال الرابع—إذا كانت الحمى محرقة مع برد الأطراف وظهر في اللسان

بثر، على ماذا يدل؟

الجواب—منقول من المقالة العاشرة من الملكي حيث يقول: هذا يدل على أن الموت قريب وذلك البثر يدل على أن في المريء والمعدة قروحاً.

السؤال الخامس—إذا كان في بدن /20a/ العليل قرحة متقدمة فأخضرت أو أسودت، على ماذا يدل[12]؟

الجواب—من المقالة العاشرة من الملكي، هذا علامة رديئة وذلك لأن المريض[13] إذا آل أمره إلى الموت فإن العضو المؤوف[14] يموت قبل كل عضو لضعف الحرارة الغريزية فيه.

السؤال السادس—إذا حدثت حمى حادة وكان باطن البدن يلتهب مع عطش وظاهره بارد، على ماذا يدل؟

الجواب—من المقالة العاشرة من الملكي، هذا دليل على الموت لأنه يدل على ورم حار في باطن البدن وأن[15] الحرارة منعكسة نحو الورم ويصير الدم إليه فيحرق[16] باطن البدن.

السؤال السابع—إذا كان بإنسان حمى حادة قوية الحرارة وسكتت الحرارة وطاب ملمس البدن من غير سبب، على ماذا يدل؟

الجواب—هذا يدل على أن الموت قريب[17] وذلك لأن الحرارة تغور إلى قعر[18] البدن فتحرق باطنه والقوّة[19] الحيوانية تثبت[20] بكليتها[21] لدفع[22] مادة المرض ولا يكون لها به طاقة فتسقط[23] القوّة[24] ويموت المريض.

السؤال الثامن—بماذا يستدل على أن /20b/ المادة قد مالت إلى أعضاء

البول حتى ينذر بأن البحران يكون به؟

الجواب—من كلّيّات القانون حيث يقول: يدل عليه[25] ثقل في المثانة[26] وإحتباس في البراز وفقدان علامات الإسهال والقيء والرعاف وحرقة في الإحليل[27] وثوران[28] البول وغلظ[29] في سائر الأيام وقد يوجد[30] الرسوب فيه.

السؤال التاسع—بماذا يستدل على أن المادة قد مالت إلى طريق البراز حتي ينذر بأن البحران يكون به؟

الجواب—من القانون لإبن سينا، يدل عليه قلة[31] البول ومغص في جميع البطن وثقل في أسفله[32] وفقدان[33] علامات القيء و[34] حدوث قراقر وإنتفاخ حالب وكثرة إنصباغ البراز وعلو ما دون الشراسيف نتوّه وإنتقال قرقرة إلى وجع الظهر[35] وقد[36] يكون النبض صغيراً مع قوّة وليس يصلب وقد يدل على البحران الإسهالي العادة في قلة الرعاف والعرق وكثرة الإختلاف وخصوصاً المعتاد شرب الماء البارد وقد[37] قيل إنه متى كان البول بعد البحران في حمى غيبية[38] أبيضاً[39] رقيقاً[40] فتوقع إختلافاً يكاد يسحج.

السؤال العاشر—بماذا يستدل على ميل /21a/ المادة إلى العروق[41] حتى ينذر بأن البحران يكون به؟

الجواب—من القانون لإبن سينا، إذا كان[42] النبض شديد الرخية[43] وكان إمساك اليد على الجلد تحصل تحته نداوة تصبغ حمرة وتجد سخونة الجلد مع ذلك أكثر مما كانت[44] وإنتفاخه وإحمراره أكثر مما كان وكان البول منصبغاً إلى غلظ وخصوصاً إذا إنصبغ في الرابع وغلظ في السابع، ولا ينبغي[45] أن يتوقع بحران عرق

مع إستطلاق من الطبيعة غالب.

السؤال الحادي عشر—بماذا يستدل على أن البحران يكون بالقيء حتى ينذر به قبل كونه؟

الجواب—من القانون إذا حدث[46] في العين ظلمة وعشاوة ومرارة فم وإختلاج شفة[47] ووجع في فم المعدة وتحلب لعاب وخفقان وإنضغاط من النبض وإنخفاض وخصوصاً إذا[48] أصاب العليل عقيب هذا نافض[49] وبرد دون الشراسيف فاحكم بأن البحران[50] واقع بالقيء لا سيّما[51] إذا كانت[52] المادة صفراوية وأصفر الوجه.

السؤال الثاني عشر—بماذا[53] يستدل على أن البحران يكون بالرعاف؟

الجواب—إذا رأى /21b/ العليل خيوطاً حمراء أو لألأ وتباريق وأحمر الوجه جداً و[54] العين و[55] الأنف وسال الدمع دفعة وشهق النبض وماج وأسرع[56] وأحتك[57] الأنف وكان إشتعال الرأس شديداً جداً والصداع ضربانياً فتوقع رعافاً لاسيّما[58] إذا دل المرض والسن والعادة والمزاج على أن المادة دموية وإن كانت[59] المادة الصفراوية [60] أيضاً، قد تبحرن[61] برعاف[62].

السؤال الثالث عشر—ما تقول في الإستسقاء الذي يكون بعقب الأمراض الحادة إذا كان معه حمى وألم، على ماذا يدل؟

الجواب—من الملكي، هذا رديء قتال وذلك أنه لما كان الإستسقاء حدوثه من برد الكبد وضعف القوّة المولدة للدم كان شفاؤه التسخين[63] وإستعمال الأدوية الحارة وكما[64] متى إستعملنا مثل هذه الأشياء زدنا في قوّة الحمى والألم وإذا[65]

كان الألم إنما يكون بسبب ورم حار وإما بسبب لذع حرارة ومتى إستعملنا الأشياء المبردة لتسكن[66] الحمى زدنا في الإستسقاء فيهلك لذلك المريض في أكثر الأحوال.

السؤال الرابع عشر—إذا رأيت بإنسان إختلاط ذهن فإذا نام وإستيقظ ثاب إليه ذهنه فإذا إستيقظ /22a/ زماناً عاد إلى إختلاطه، على ماذا يدل؟

الجواب—من الملكي، هذه دلالة[67] محمودة لأن الطبيعة في وقت النوم تكون قد قهرت مادة المرض وأنضجتها بقوّتها إلا أنه ينبغي أن يعلم أنه ليس في كل علة جودة الذهن علامة جيدة لأن أصحاب النزف[68] وأصحاب السل يهلكون وذهنهم سليم لكن في الأمراض الحادة وأمراض الرأس.

السؤال الخامس عشر—إذا حدث بصاحب السرسام عطاس، على ماذا يدل؟

الجواب—من الملكي، هذا دليل محمود وذلك أن الدماغ وبطونه[69] قد قوي على دفع الفضل والشئ المؤذي ولذلك قال جالينوس في العلل والأعراض: إن[70] العطاس إذا لم يكن عن زكام كان من أنفع الأشياء للرأس المملوء بخاراً إلا أنه مذموم في سائر أمراض الصدر لأنه يزعج[71] الصدر ويحدر إليه مادة.

السؤال السادس عشر—إذا خرج في البراز حيات في يوم من أيام البحران، على ماذا يدل؟

الجواب—من الملكي، هذا دليل محمود[72] لأن الطبيعة تكون قد قويت على دفع المادة المؤذية فإندفعت الحيات مع ما دفعت بقوّتها/22b/.

السؤال السابع عشر—إذا رأيت بإنسان صمماً[73] وقد حدث بعقبه[74] حمى حادة فأصابه إسهال مري، على ماذا يدل؟

الجواب—إن هذا الصمم يحدث عن تراقي المرار إلى الرأس فإذا إنحدر ذلك المرار[75] إلى أسفل إنقضى الصمم وكذلك[76] إذا[77] كان بإنسان صمم إنقطع ذلك الإختلاف والقضية[78] في هذا ضدها فيما قبله[79] .

السؤال الثامن عشر—في أي المواضع تكون البواسير إذا ظهرت دليلاً محموداً؟

الجواب—قال صاحب الملكي، إذا حدث بأصحاب الوسواس السوداوي[80] والسرسام البواسير كان ذلك دليلاً محموداً وذلك بسبب إنحدار المادة من العلو إلى السفل[81] .

السؤال التاسع عشر—إذا حدث بمن به حمى محرقة نافض في يوم من أيام البحران، ما دلالته؟

الجواب—من الملكي، هذا يدل على إنقضائها وذلك لأن الحمى المطبقة تكون من الخلط العفن داخل الأوردة والعروق والنافض يكون حدوثه عند خروج ذلك الخلط عن الأوردة والعروق وإنصبابه إلى الأعضاء الحساسة.

السؤال العشرون—كيف تقضي بالسلامة من ذات الجنب أو ذات الرئة من جهة ما ينفث؟

الجواب—/23a/من الملكي، إذا كان ما ينفث في إبتداء المرض رقيقاً أبيض ثم يغلظ بعد قليل بسهولة من غير شدة[82] ودفعه بقوّة وهو ليس بأسود

ولا أخضر ولا أصفر ولم تكن له رائحة، دل ذلك على نضج المرض والسلامة منه وقصر مدته.

الباب الخامس في الأدوية وهو عشرون مسألة

السؤال الأول—إذا تركبت حرارة معتدلة مع جوهر غليظ لطيف أو مع جوهر متوسط، كيف يكون الطعم؟

الجواب—من المقالة الثانية من الأصول لإبن رضوان حيث يقول: الحرارة المعتدلة له مع الجوهر الغليظ تحدث الطعم الحلو و مع الجوهر اللطيف تحدث الطعم الدسم و مع المتوسط تحدث الطعم التفه.

السؤال الثاني—إذا تركبت البرودة مع الجوهر اللطيف أو مع الجوهر الغليظ أو مع الجوهر المتوسط، كيف يكون الطعم؟

الجواب—من المقالة الثانية من كتاب الأصول لإبن رضوان، إذا تركبت البرودة مع الجوهر الغليظ حدث الطعم العفص فإن تركبت مع الجوهر اللطيف حدث الطعم الحامض وإن تركبت مع المتوسط حدث الطعم القابض.

السؤال الثالث—إذا تركبت حرارة زائدة مع جوهر/23b/ غليظ أو لطيف أو متوسط، كيف يكون الطعم؟

الجواب—من كتاب الأصول لإبن رضوان، إن تركبت حرارة زائدة مع جوهر غليظ كان الطعم مراً[1] فإن تركبت حرارة زائدة مع جوهر لطيف كان الطعم حريفاً وإن تركبت حرارة زائدة مع جوهر متوسط كان الطعم مالحاً.

السؤال الرابع—إلى كم قسم تقسم الأمنان الساقطة وكم عددها ومن أين تجلب كل واحد منها؟

الجواب—من المقالة الحادية عشر من المرشد للتميمي حيث يقول: أما أقسامها فقسمان، أحدهما ضرب[2] من الأهوية على الأشجار فمنها قابض الطعم كالكشوث ومنها حادة القوّة كالأفثيمون ومنها مر يسير المرارة[3] عطري كالورس الهندي والحبشي واليماني، والقنبيل، واللاذن، واللك فهذا هو قسم الأدوية الهوائية الساقطة على الأشجار[4] وأما القسم الثاني من الأمنان وهو جوهر من الحلاوات التي تخل[5] بالماء والنار[6] وتجمد ببرد الهواء كالترنجبين والعسل وأما عددها فخمسة عشر، العسل، وسكر العشر، والترنجبين، والكزنكبين، ـــ[7]، والشرخست[8] ، والمن، والشمع، واللاذن[9] ، واللك، والورس، والقنبيل، والكشوث، والأفثيمون، والسكر، فالعسل، قال التميمي في /24a/ مرشده هو من يسقط من الهواء بكل بلد وبكل إقليم من الأمصار المسكونة وغير المسكونة وسقوطه على ورق أنواع من الأزهار والأنوار[10]، وأما سكر العشر فهو من يسقط على ورق العشر رطباً كسقوط الأندية على النبات فيكتسب من ورق العشر قوّة مطلقة للطبيعة ويجمد على الورق، وأما الترنجبين فهو من يقع على شوك الشبرق[11] وفيه ثمر الشبرق موجود فيه مثل الماش وهو بأرض خراسان، وأما الكزنكبين فهو من يقع بخراسان على ورق الطرفاء والأثل، وأما ـــ[12] فهو من يقع على ورق الخلاف، وأما الشرخست[13] فهو من يسقط بهراة[14] على صنف من الشوك البارد المزاج، وأما المن نفسه فهو يسقط على جلنار المظ وورقه

وهو الرمان البري وعلى ورق السدر والخوخ والبلوط باليمن، أما الشمع فالأطباء مجمعون على أنه من يقول التميمي في مرشده، أما أنا فلست أرى ذلك بل أرى أن الشمع جسم قفري يتكون من ريق النحل، ويخرج[15] من بطونها كمثل ما يتكون القز من ريق دود القز والدليل عليه ما تراه ينتقل فيه من إختلاف ألوانه مع سن النحل عاماً بعد عام وذلك أنا نرى الشمع ينتقل مع سن النحل[16] في كل عام يأتي عليه إلى لون غير لونه الأول فمن ذلك أنا نجد /24b/ شمع الفراخ المسماة طرود أول عام أبيض نقياً[17] وثاني سنة يتغير إلى الصفرة و ثالث سنة يكون أقوى صفرة ورابع سنة يكون أحمر وخامس سنة يكون أشد حمرة وسادس سنة يضرب إلى السواد وسابع سنة يكون أسود شديد السواد وهو غاية ما يعمر النحل، وأما اللاذن فهو من الأمنان الساقطة مثل الطل وأكثر مسقطه هو بجزيرة قبرس على شجر يرتعيه أغنام تلك الجزيرة فإذا رعت الغنم ورق ذلك النبت ووطئته بأظلافها تعلق بشعور لحاها وبأظلافها وتكاثف بعضه على بعض حتى يصير مثل الكعك[18] الذي يسمى الزوفا الرطب المتعلق بلوايا الضأن فيجمع اللاذن من شعور تلك الأغنام بأمشاط الحديد وديسقوريدوس يقول إنه من[19] يقع على صنف من الشجر يقال له قسوس فإذا رعت الغنم تعلق في لحاها وأظلافها لأنه في كيان الدبق، أما اللك فقوم قالوا إنه صمغ وليس بصحيح والدليل على أنه من الأمنان[20] أنا نجده ملبساً بقضبان الكرم التي يكون منها الورق والعنب فنجد العود المركب عليه اللك في غلظ الأصبع[21] الخنصر بل دونها بكثير ونجد ما قد علا عليه من اللك[22] يربو ويزيد

على غلظ القضيب الحامل له أضعافاً كثيرة حتى يكون في غلظ الإبهام وأغلظ وليس في قضبان الكرم من اللدونة الصمغية /25a/ ما أن يغلظ ذلك العود الدقيق فيلبسه ويتراكب[23] عليه فدل ذلك على أنه جسم لطيف هوائي يسقط[24] على ظاهر تلك القضبان فتعلقه[25] بالخاصية التي جعلت فيها وهو مختص[26] بموضعين من الهند أحدهما الديبل[27] والآخر الصمرة أو سندان، وأما الورس فيسمى الحص والقنديد[28] وهو عند قوم الورس الحبشي وليس ينبت ببلاد الحبشة فقط بل قد يسقط بالصين ويجلب من الصين[29] إلى الهند ويسمى[30] الورس الهندي وقد يسقط أيضاً ببلاد اليمن وهو ثلاثة أصناف أحدها يسقط بالصين و يجلب إلى الهند، الثاني الحبشي وهو يسقط ببلاد الحبشة ويجلب إلى مكة، الثالث اليماني وهو ما يسقط بأودية اليمن ويجلب منها وسقوطه على صنف من الشجر يشاكل الباذروج ويشاكل ورقه وزهره، أما القنبيل فهو أحد الأمنان الساقطة وسقوطه يكون بأودية اليمن كسقوط الورس، وأما الكشوث بأرض العراق ويسقط[31] على كل شئ يشاكل الباذروج وهو الحوك، وأما الأفثيمون فهو أحد الأمنان الساقطة من الهواء[32] وهو يسقط على صنف من الصعاتر يسمى الصعتيرة وهو ثلاثة أصناف من ثلاثة أمصار فأفضله ما يجيء من جزيرة إقريطش وهو ما يجيء من البيت المقدس أو من ضياع فلسطين، أما السكر فقوم يرون أنه من الأمنان الساقطة من الهواء لكنه أحد العصارات المتخذة بالجمد.

/25b/ **السؤال الخامس**—كم هي الأقفار التي تخرج من بطن الأرض؟

الجواب—ثمانية أصناف وهو في[33] المقالة الحادية عشر من المرشد

للتميمي وهو العنبر والسندروس والموميا الفارسي والموميا المغربي وقفر اليهود والقار العراقي والنفط والكبريت.

السؤال السادس—ما تقول في ثمر الطرفاء هل ذكر أحد أن له فائدة في الجذام وإن كان ذلك فما علته؟

الجواب—من الأدوية المفردة لإبن وافد حيث يقول: أخبرني ثقة أن إمرأة ظهر عليها الجذام فسقيت من طبيخ أصول الطرفاء والزبيب مرارا[34] فبرئت[35] وأنه جربه مرة أخرى فصح. قال إبن وافد: وأنا أقول علته[36] ذلك أن[37] علة هاؤلاء كانت عن ورم الطحال أو سدة فيه إمتنع بسبب أحدهما جذب الخلط السودائي[38] من الدم وتصفيته عنه وكان ذلك سبباً لظهور الداء فيهم فلما تحلل الورم[39] إنفتحت السدة بإستعمالهم هذا الدواء[40] بما في طبعه من التقطيع والجلاء فعادوا إلى الصحة.

السؤال السابع—ما تقول في الحصى المتولد في مثانة الإنسان؟ هل ذكر له نفع في مرض من الأمراض أم لا؟

الجواب—من المقالة الثانية عشر من المرشد للتميمي حيث يقول: إن الحجر المتولد في المثانة إذا سحق وكحلت منه العين الكائن فيها البياض جلاه وأزاله /26a/ بقوّة.

السؤال الثامن—ما هو[41] الداء الذي إذا يشرب الإنسان فيه بوله لنفسه إنتفع به؟

الجواب—من الأدوية المفردة لإبن وافد حيث يقول: بول الإنسان إذا شربه

صاحبه نفع من نهشة[42] الأفعى والأدوية القتالة وإبتداء الحبن.

السؤال التاسع—ما الذي ذكر في السمن من المنفعة الغريبة وما كيفية العمل به؟

الجواب—من المرشد للتميمي حيث يقول: إن السمن من خاصيته أن يوقف العلة المسماة داء الأسد وهو الجذام وذلك أن يغلى ويسكب في أبزن واسع أو قدر ويترك[43] حتى يمكن أن يجلس فيه ثم جلس فيه صاحب العلة غارقاً إلى حلقه ويسكب منه على[44] رأسه دائماً إلى أن يبرد ثم أخرج[45] منه وإغتسل بالماء الحار ثم لبس[46] ثيابه فإنه متى لزم هذا الفعل أسبوعاً أوقف العلة عنه ذلك الحول كله ولم يزد[47] لكنه في العام المقبل يحتاج أن يعاود ذلك الفعل.

السؤال العاشر—ما الذي ذكر في لبن الكلبة من المنافع؟

الجواب—من المرشد للتميمي حيث يقول: إن لبن الكلبة الفتية السن إذا طلي به موضع الشعر الزائدة في باطن الجفن ثم طلي منه على مواضعه لم يعد ينبت فيه شعر أبداً وكذلك في سائر الجسد بعد نتفه وإن طلي منه على منابت أسنان /26b/ الأطفال ولثاتهم الوارمة عند خروج أسنانهم سكن الوجع وأسرع بخروج أسنان الأطفال[48] بغير وجع ويخرج الجنين الميت إذا تحمل منه.

السؤال الحادي عشر—ما الفائدة المذكورة في قلب نوى الزيتون وفي صمغه؟

الجواب—من المرشد للتميمي حيث يقول: وأما القلب الموجود في جوف نوى الزيتون فإنه إذا سحق وخلط بشحم ودقيق وعمل منه ضماد قلع البياض

العارض للأظفار وأما صمغه فقال حبيش: إنه[49] إذا سحق وذر منه على الجراحة ألحمها.

السؤال الثاني عشر—كم هي الأدوية التي ذكر إبن وافد أنها حارة يابسة في الدرجة الأولى وما هي؟

الجواب—من كتاب الأدوية المفردة لإبن وافد، أما عدتها فإثنان وستون وهي أفسنتين، أرز، أنزروت، إسفنج[50]، أُسطوخودس[51]، إكليل الملك، إذخر[52]، أبل[53]، بزر كتان، بابونج[54]، بادرنجوية[55]، داذي[56]، دوسر، دار شيشعان، هرنوة[57]، حرير، حنطة، حور[58]، طرفاء، كرنب[59]، كرسنة، كزبرة، كرم وعنب[60]، كشوث[61]، كلابي[62]، لبلاب، لاذن، لوف، محلب، من، ميعة[63]، نيلنج[64]، نشارة[65]، بنجكشت[66]، نارمشك، /27a/ سكر، سنبل، سادج، سك[67]، سرو، سرخس[68]، سندروس، سنا، فستق[69]، فوة، فاونياقو[70]، صنوبر، قاقلى، قطن، قلت[71]، قنبيل، رطب[72]، شيلم[73]، شاهسفرم[74]، نرجس[75]، خندروس[76]، خطمي، غافت، غاريقون، قاقلة[77]، ترمس.

السؤال الثالث عشر—كم هي الأدوية التي ذكرها إبن وافد في كتابه أنها حارة رطبة في الأولى؟

الجواب—ثلاثة عشر، جوز، حندم[78]، حمص، لوبيا، لوز، لسان ثور[79]، ملوخ[80]، سمسم، عناب، قصب، شقاقل، خصى الثعلب، خصى الكلب.

السؤال الرابع عشر—كم هي الأدوية الباردة اليابسة في الدرجة الأولى؟

الجواب—من كتاب الأدوية المفردة[81] لإبن وافد، أربعة وأربعون وهي خمسة وأربعون، آس، أُشنة، أقاقيا، أملج[82]، أسطير أطيقوس[83]، باقلا، بلوط،

باذاورد، بسد، بردي[84]، جاورس، ديس، دخن[86]، دردار، دبساقوس[87]، هليلج، ورد، زعرور، حناء، /27b/ حماض، حسك، حزاز الصخر[87]، كمثرى، لحية التيس، ماش، مقل[88]، نخلة[89]، سدر[90]، سادروان[91]، سلت، علس، عليق[92]، قرطمان، قاتل أبيه، قصب، رمان، شكاعا، شعير، توت، تفاح، سفرجل، خل، خرنوب، خلاف، غرا[93].

السؤال الخامس عشر—كم هي الأدوية الباردة الرطبة في الدرجة الأولى التي ذكرها إبن وافد في مفرداته؟

الجواب—أحد عشر، إجاص، إسفاناخ[94]، دلب، بنفسج[95]، هندبا، نوفر[96]، قراصيا[97]، قطف، سوس، سلق، خبازا[98].

السؤال السادس عشر—كم هي الأدوية التي ذكر إبن وافد أنها حارة يابسة في الدرجة الثانية؟

الجواب—أحد وستون، أنجرة، أظفار[99]، أبنوس[100]، ـــ[101]، أناغلس[102]، الأسفاقس[103]، فرنجمشك[104]، باذروج، بهار، بطم بلسان، جوز بوا، جوز، جلوز[105]، جوز الرقع، جعدة، جزر، دبق، وسخ الكوائر[106]، ورس، زراوند، زرنباد، زعفران، حلبة، حماحم[107]، ياسمين، كفر[108] اليهود، جندبيدستر[109]، /28a/ كندر، كمافيطوس[110]، كمادريوس، لك مو، مصطكي[111]، مري، مسك، بنك، نسرين، نرجس، سوسن، سلجم، سعد[112]، سقولوفندريون[113]، سورنجان، عسل، عنبر، عود، فراسيون، فلنجة، فاغرة[114]، صبر، قرطم، قلقاس، قثاء الحمار، قصب الذريرة، راوند[115]، شهدانج، تين، خيري، خنثى، خروع.

السؤال السابع عشر—كم هي الأدوية الحارة الرطبة في الدرجة الثانية التي ذكرها إبن وافد؟

الجواب—ستة، بهمن[116]، جرجير، حب القلقل، لسان العصفور[117]، مغاث[118]، نارجيل.

السؤال الثامن عشر—كم هي الأدوية الباردة اليابسة في الدرجة الثانية التي ذكرها إبن وافد؟

الجواب—ثلاثة عشر، أمير باريس[119]، بزر قطونا، جلنار، كثيراء[120]، لسان الحمل، ماميثا، سماق، عوسج، عفص، عنب الثعلب، صمغ[121]، رامك، ريباس.

السؤال التاسع عشر—/28b/كم هي الأدوية الباردة الرطبة في الدرجة الثانية التي ذكرها إبن وافد؟

الجواب—تسعة، بقلة يمانية، بطيخ، وقثاء، وحناء[122]، دلاع، طحلب، كمأة، مشمش، قرع، خس، خوخ.

السؤال العشرون—كم هي الأدوية المفردة[123] الحارة اليابسة في الدرجة الثالثة والحارة الرطبة والباردة اليابسة فيها والباردة الرطبة؟

الجواب—أما الأدوية الحارة اليابسة في الدرجة الثالثة من كتاب إبن وافد فعدتها ثلاثة وثمانون[124]، أنجدان[125]، أنيسون، أقحوان، أسارون، أبهل، أفثيمون[126]، أُشنان، بسفانج[127]، بخور مريم، بوزيدان، بل وفل وشل[128]، جاوشير[129]، جنطيانا، دخان[130]، دوقوا[131]، دار صيني، هيوفاريقون، وشق، وج[132]، زرنب، زفت، حرشف[133]، حامالاون[134] لوقس[135]، مالس[136]، جوز رومي[137]، حب الرأس، حب البان[138]، حماما[139]،

حب عرعر، حاشاء، حنظل، حب النيل[140]، خاما أقطي[141]، حرمل، يربطورة[142]، كمون، كبابة، كراويا[143]، كرفس، كسرم[144]، موميا[145]، مقل اليهود، مروية، ينبوت[146]، مرزنجوش، نانخواة، نعنع، نمام، سذاب، /29a/سليخة، سكبينج، سقمونيا، عنصل، عكوب، عروق[147]، فجل، أنافس، إسقلينوس[148]، بنجنكشت[149]، فوتنج[150]، قلفونية[151]،صعتر، قنطوريون كبير[152]، قنطوريون[153] دقيق[154]، قردمانا، قيصوم، قسط[155]، قرنفل،قنة، قرمز، قبيطون[156]، قرة العين، رازيانج، شبث، شجرة مريم، شونيز، شيح، تربد، ثوم، خولنجان[157]، خربقان، غار، درونج[158]، زوفا، راتينج. وأما الحارة الرطبة في الدرجة الثالثة فأربعة وهي زنجبيل، حب الزلم[159]، راسن، تافسيا. وأما الباردة اليابسة في الدرجة الثالثة فتسع، بنج، دم الأخوين، يبروح، كافور، فوفل، صندل، شوكران، تمرهندي، طباشير. وأما الباردة الرطبة في الدرجة الثالثة فأربع، بقلة حمقاء، حي العالم، عصى[160] الراعي، فطر.

الباب السادس في المداواة وهو عشرون مسألة

السؤال الأول—كم هي الأعراض المقصودة في المعالجة وما الذي يرشد إليها؟

الجواب—من الكتاب التاسع والخمسين /29b/ من الكتب المائة للمسيحي حيث يقول: إنها خمسة، أحدها العرض[1] الذي يقصد نحو كيفية الشئ الذي به يكون[2] المعالجة[3] ويرشد لذلك نوع المرض. الثاني العرض الذي يقصد به نحو مقدار الشئ الذي به يكون المعالجة والذي يرشد إلى[4] ذلك[5] هو مزاج البدن ومقدار المرض وحال سائر الأشياء التي تدل[6] بمخالفتها وموافقتها. الثالث العرض الذي به يقصد نحو الوقت الذي فيه يستعمل الشئ الذي يكون به المعالجة والذي يرشد إلى ذلك هو الوقت[7] من المرض ومقدار قوّة المرض وحال سائر الأشياء التي تدل بموافقتها ومخالفتها. الرابع العرض الذي يقصد به نحو الوجه في إستعمال الشئ الذي يكون به المعالجة. الخامس العرض الذي يقصد به نحو إختيار مادة الشئ الذي يكون به المعالجة والذي يرشد إلى هذين العرضين[8] هو المرض والمزاج والقوّة وسائر الأشياء التي تدل بموافقتها ومخالفتها وهي البلد والوقت الحاضر وحال الهواء[9].

السؤال الثاني—كم هي طرق معالجة الأمراض في كل واحد من الأعضاء

خاصة وكيف هي؟

الجواب—من الكتاب التاسع والخمسين من الكتب[10] المائة للمسيحي، أربعة، أولها الطريق المأخوذ من مزاج العضو العليل، الثاني الطريق المأخوذ من خلقته، الثالث الطريق المأخوذ /30a/ من وضعه، الرابع الطريق المأخوذ من قوّته. أما المأخوذ من مزاج العضو العليل فمثل أن الأعضاء كلما غلبت فيه الحرارة كاللحم أو غلبت فيه البرودة كالعصب أو كان متوسطاً كالجلد صار كل واحد منها إذا تغير مزاجه الطبيعي يحتاج إلى ردة إليه بالأشياء المائلة عن الإعتدال إلى خلاف الوجه الذي مال إليه. وأما المأخوذ من خلقة العضو فإن من الأعضاء ما هو مجوف كالمعدة ومنها غير مجوف ومنها مصمت بمنزلة[11] أعصاب اليدين والرجلين ومنها ما لها تجويف من داخل وخارج معاً بمنزلة الرئة فإنها تحيط بها الصدر من خارج ومن داخل أقسام قصبة الرئة والعروق الضوارب متفرقة فيها فمتى كان العضو سحيقاً متخلخلاً كالرئة لم يحتمل أن يداوي بأدوية قوية ومتى كان كثيفاً ملززاً كالكليتين إحتمل أدوية قوية ومتى كان متوسطاً كالكبد إحتاج إلى دواء متوسط. وأما المأخوذ من وضع العضو فهو أن ينظر الموضع الذي فيه العضو في معالجة سوء مزاجه لأنه إن كان قريب الموضع حتى يمكن الدواء أن يلاقيه و قوّة الدواء باقية على حالها أو كان بعيداً لا يمكن الدواء أن يصل إليه حتى يمر بأعضاء آخر زدنا[12] في مقدار الدواء بمقدار ما نعلم أنه ينقص/30b/ من قوّته في الطريق قبل الوصول إليه. أما الطريق المأخود من قوّة العضو فهو أن يعتبر هل يفعل فعلاً عامياً ينتفع به في جميع البدن مثل المعدة والحجاب وأن يعتبر هل ذكي

الحس بمنزلة العين ومتى إحتجنا أن نداوي[13] الكبد والمعدة بضماد محلل خلطنا مع الأدوية المحللة أدوية قابضة طيبة الرائحة لتبقى قوّة الدواء على ما هي عليه.

السؤال الثالث—كم هي مراتب المعالجة بالدواء؟

الجواب—من كلّيّات القانون، ثلاثة. أحدها قانون إختيار كيفيته أي[14] إختياره حاراً أو بارداً أو رطباً أو يابساً. الثاني قانون إختيار كميته وهذا ينقسم إلى قانون تقدير وزنه وإلى قانون تقدير كيفيته. الثالث قانون ترتيب وقته.

السؤال الرابع—كم هي الشرائط التي تراعي[15] في الجذب؟

الجواب—من كلّيّات القانون، أربعة. الأول مخالفة الجهة كما تجذب[16] من اليمين إلى اليسار ومن فوق إلى أسفل. الثاني مراعاة المشاركة كما يحتبس[17] الطمث يوضع المحاجم على[18] الثديين[19] جذباً إلى الشريك. الثالث مراعاة المحاذاة كما يفصد في علل الكبد الباسليق الأيمن وفي علل الطحال الباسليق الأيسر. الرابع مراعاة البعيد[20] في ذلك لئلا /31a/ يكون المجذوب إليه قريباً من المجذوب منه.

السؤال الخامس—كم هي الخلال[21] المحوجة إلى تركيب الأدوية وما مثالها؟

الجواب—من الفصول للرازي، خمسة. أحدها أنه ربما كان الدواء الذي ينفع من علة ما و[22] يقوى عضواً ما يضر[23] بآخر فيضطر معه إلى تركيب[24] ما يمنع من ذلك، مثال ذلك إخلاطنا[25] الجندبيدستر بالأفيون لئلا يعظم ضرره[26]. الثاني إن يكون الدواء لا يصل إلى الموضع الذي نريد فنضطر إلى[27] أن نخلط معه[28] ما يوصله إليه كإخلاطنا[29] الأفاوية اللطيفة بالطين المختوم والصمغ[30] عند نفث الدم من الرئة والصدر. الثالث إن تكون أدوية نافعة لعلة ما إلا أن بعضها أنفع

من بعض لبعض الأبدان والأمزاج[31] فيريد الطبيب أن يكون عنده دواء يصلح لتلك العلة في أكثر الأمر و[32] يريد الطبيب أن يكون عنده دواء يصلح أن يستعمله[33] في علل كثيرة فيضطر لتركيب[34] ذلك الدواء من أدوية نافعة لعلل شتى كالترياق مثلاً النافع من أدواء شتى[35]. الرابع أنه ربما إحتاج إلى[36] أن يخرج من البدن أخلاطاً مختلفة فيحتاج أن يركب ذلك الدواء من أدوية كل واحد منها يخرج خلطاً من الأخلاط مثال ذلك حب جالينوس المعروف بالقوقايا المركب من الصبر والسقمونيا /31b/ وشحم الحنظل وعصارة الأفسنتين. الخامس أنه ربما كان[37] الدواء النافع لا[38] تستعمل[39] حتى يحل بشيء آخر[40] كالمرداسنج وسائر الأدوية الحجرية التي لا يمكن أن يستعمل[41] في[42] المراهم حتى تحل[43] بالأدهان والخلول وتركب وتذاب[44] مع الصموغ والشحوم.

السؤال السادس—كم هي أصناف معالجة سوء المزاج؟

الجواب—من كلّيّات القانون، ثلاثة. أحدها إن يكون سوء المزاج مستحكماً[45] فيكون علاجه بالضد على الإطلاق وهذا هو المداواة المطلقة. الثاني، أما إن يكون حد الكون[46] فإصلاحه ومداواته[47] مع التقدم بالحفظ يمنع[48] السبب. الثالث، وأما إن يريد أن يكون ويحتاج فيه إلى منع السبب فقط ويسمى التقدم بالحفظ.

السؤال السابع—كم هي الأشياء التي تدل على صواب الحكم في الإستفراغ؟

الجواب—من كلّيّات القانون، عشرة. الإمتلاء، والقوّة[49]، والمزاج، والأعراض الملائحة[50]، والسحنة، والسن، والفصل[51]، وحال هواء البلد[52]،

وعادة الإستفراغ، والصناعة.

السؤال الثامن—كم هي الأمور التي تقصد في كل إستفراغ؟

الجواب—من كلّيّات القانون، خمسة. أحدها إستفراغ ما يجب إستفراغه ويعقبه[53] /32a/ لا محالة راحة. الثاني، تأمل جهة ميله كالغثيان ينقى بالقيء والمغص بالإسهال. الثالث، عضو مخرجه من جهة ميله كالباسليق الأيمن لعلل الكبد لا القيفال الأيمن فإنه إن أخطئ في هذا فربما[54] جلب خطراً وينبغي[55] أن يكون عضو المخرج أخس[56] لئلا تميل المادة إلى ما هو أشرف ويجب أن يكون مخرجه منه طبيعياً كأعضاء البول لحدبة الكبد والأمعاء لتقعيره وربما كان العضو الذي يتدفع[57] منه هو العضو الذي يجب أن يستفرغ منه لكن به علة فيحتاج أن يمال إلى غيره. الرابع، وقت إستفراغه وجالينوس يحزم[58] القول بأن الأمراض المزمنة ينتظر فيها النضج قبل الإستفراغ وبعد النضج[59] يجب[60] أن يسقي من[61] الملطفات. وأما في الأمراض الحادة فالأصوب أيضاً إنتظار النضج وخصوصاً إن كانت ساكنة. وأما إن كانت متحركة فالمبادرة[62] إلى إستفراغ المادة أولا[63] إذ ضرر حركتها أكثر من ضرر إستفراغها قبل نضجها وخصوصاً إذا كانت الأخلاط رقيقة وخصوصاً إذا كانت في تجاويف العروق غير مداخلة[64] للأعضاء. وأما إذا كان الخلط محصوراً في عضو فلا تحرك[65] البتة حتى ينضج ويحصل له القوام المعتدل.

السؤال التاسع—إذا إجتمعت أمراض فبأي المعالجات تبتدئ؟

الجواب—من الكلّيّات، تبتدئ بما يخصه إحدى[66] الخواص /32b/ الثلاث، أحدها بالذي لا يبرأ الثاني[67] دون[68] بروءه[69] مثل الورم والقرحة إذا إجتمعا فإنا

نعالج الورم أولاً حتى يزول[70] المزاج الذي يصحبه ولا يمكن أن يبرأ معه القرحة ثم نعالج القرحة. الثاني[71]، إن يكون أحدهما هو السبب في الثاني مثل أنه إذا عرضت سدة وحمى عالجنا السدة أولاً ثم الحمى ولم نبال من الحمى لأن الحمى يستحيل أن تزول وسببها باقٍ وعلاجها[72] التجفيف وهو يضر بالحمى. الثالث[73]، إن يكون أحدهما أشد إهتماماً كما لو[74] إجتمع سونوخس وفالج[75] فإنا نعالج سونوخس[76] بالتطفيئة والفصد ولا نلتفت إلى الفالج. وأما إذا إجتمع المرض والعرض فإنا نبتدي بعلاج المرض[77] إلا أن يغلب[78] العرض فحينئذ نقصد[79] العرض ولا نلتفت إلى المرض[80] كما نسقي المخدرات في القولنج الشديد الوجع إذا صعب وإن كان يضر[81] نفس القولنج.

السؤال العاشر—كم هي[82] منافع السكنجبين؟

الجواب—من تجارب إبن المدور نقلة من مقالة حنين في السكنجبين، وهي ثمانية وثمانون منفعة، الأول أنه يبرد المزاج المائل إلى الحرارة المفرطة ويعدله بتطفيئة تلك الحرارة وتهديته لها. الثاني أنه يحمى البدن البارد إذا شرب صرفاً. الثالث أنه يرطب البدن اليابس إذا شرب بمزاج كثير يكون هو الربع والماء ثلاثة أرباع. الرابع أنه يجفف البدن الرطب بتقطيعه الرطوبات /33a/ وإحدارها من البدن ونفضها إلى خارج إذا شرب صرفاً وخاصة إذا كان سخناً. الخامس أنه ينفع من الغب الدائرة. السادس أنه ينفع من الغب الدائمة. السابع أنه ينفع من حمى الربع النائبة. الثامن أنه ينفع من حمى الدق. التاسع أنه ينفع من الحمى المواظبة الدائمة. العاشر، ينفع من الحمى المواظبة النائبة. الحادي عشر، ينفع

من الحمى المطبقة المعروفة بسونوخس وهي الدموية. الثاني عشر، ينفع من الحمى المحرقة. الثالث عشر، ينفع من الحمي المركبة من حمى بلغم وحمى غب دائمة.

الرابع عشر، ينفع من حمى مركبة من حمى بلغمية دائمة وحمى بلغمية نائبة.

الخامس عشر، ينفع[83] من حمى مركبة من غب دائمة وغب نائبة. السادس عشر، ينفع من الحمى المركبة من حمى[84] بلغم دائمة وغب نائبة وهي شطر الغب. الثامن عشر، ينفع من تركيب [حمى] غب نائبة وحمى ربع. التاسع عشر، ينفع من تركيب حمى ربع نائبة وربع دائمة. العشرون، ينفع من تركيب حمى غب دائمة وربع دائمة. الحادي والعشرون، ينفع من تركيب حمى غب دائمة وربع نائبة. الثاني والعشرون، ينفع من تركيب حمى غب نائبة وربع دائمة. الثالث والعشرون، ينفع من تركيب حمى غب نائبة ذات[85] فترات وبلغمية ذات فترات وربع ذات فترات. الرابع والعشرون، ينفع من /33b/ تركيب بلغمية ذات فترات وغب ذات فترات.

الخامس والعشرون، ينفع من تركيب حمى بلغمية دائمة وربع ذات فترات. الثامن والعشرون، ينفع من حمى عفونه الأخلاط بأسرها ويخللها ويجلوها. التاسع والعشرون، ينفع من حمى الدق التي يكون حدوثها في الرطوبة التي في[86] الأعضاء الباطنة. الثلاثون، ينفع من حمى الدق التي يكون[87] حدوثها في الأعضاء الرطبة. الحادي والثلاثون، ينفع من حمى الدق التي يكون حدوثها في الرطوبة الموجودة في نفس الأعضاء الأصلية. الثاني والثلاثون، ينفع من حمى يوم الحادثة عن التعب. الثالث والثلاثون، ينفع[88] من حمى يوم الحادثة عن السكر. الرابع والثلاثون، ينفع من حمى يوم الحادثة عن التخمة. الخامس والثلاثون، ينفع من حمى يوم الحادثة

عن البرد الشديد. السادس والثلاثون، ينفع من حمى يوم الحادثة عن إحتراق الشمس وشدة السموم الصيفية. السابع والثلاثون، ينفع من حمى يوم الحادثة عن تكاثف ظاهر البدن كما يحدث لمن[89] يستحمر بها الشب. الثامن والثلاثون، ينفع من الحمى الحادثة عن الأرق الحادث بسبب الحزن. التاسع والثلاثون، ينفع[90] من حمى يوم الحادثة من الهم والغم. الأربعون، ينفع[91] من حمى يوم الحادثة عن السهر الذي لا يعرف له سبب. الحادي والأربعون، ينفع[92] من حمى يوم الحادثة للعاشق /34a/ أو من كلام مؤلم أو هَجر[93]. الثاني والأربعون، ينفع من سائر الحميات المخلطة[94]. الثالث والأربعون، ينفع من الغشي الحادث من الإمتلاء الذي يسد الطبقات. الرابع والأربعون، ينفع من الغشي الحادث من سوء مزاج[95]. الخامس والأربعون، ينفع من الغشي الحادث من الوجع. السادس والأربعون، ينفع من إختناق الرحم. السابع والأربعون، ينفع من السكتة والإغماء إذا يغرغر به صرفاً ودلك به الحلق مع إيارج فيقرا[96]. الثامن والأربعون، ينفع من اللذع العارض في المعدة. التاسع والأربعون، ينفع من الغشي الحادث في إبتداء نوبة الحمى. الخمسون، ينفع من السرسام. الحادي والخمسون، ينفع من البرسام. الثاني والخمسون، ينفع من ذات الجنب. الثالث والخمسون، ينفع من ذات الرئة. الرابع والخمسون، ينفع من الصداع الحادث من الشمس. الخامس والخمسون، ينفع من الصداع الحادث من الرياح ومن سوء مزاج حار مخالط لمادة. السادس والخمسون، ينفع من الصداع الحادث من سوء مزاج بارد مخالط لمادة. السابع والخمسون، ينفع من الصداع الحادث من الرياح الباردة. الثامن والخمسون،

ينفع من الصداع /34b/ الحادث عن شرب الخمر والخمار. التاسع والخمسون، ينفع من السدر والدوار. الستون، ينفع من الصداع التابع لألم فم المعدة. الحادي والستون، ينفع من الشقيقة المزمنة والحادة. الثاني والستون، ينفع من قرانيطس[97]. الثالث والستون، ينفع من ألم الدماغ من الخلط المحترق[98] والسوداوي[99]. الرابع والستون، ينفع من الإختلاج[100] إذا كان صرفاً. الخامس والستون، ينفع من السعال الحادث عن الرطوبة إذا كان صرفا[101]. السادس والستون، ينفع من السدد الحادثة في العروق التي بين الكبد والمرارة. السابع والستون، يفتح المجاري التي بين الكبد والمرارة[102]. الثامن والستون، يفتح المجاري التي بين الكبد والطحال. التاسع والستون، يفتح المجاري التي بين المعدة والمرارة[103]. السبعون، ينفع من أنواع الإستسقاء خصوصاً اللحمي. الحادي والسبعون، يفتت حصاة الكلى إذا شرب صرفاً مع رماد العقارب. الثاني والسبعون، ينفع من الماشرا. الثالث والسبعون، ينفع من الدماميل العارضة في البدن. الرابع والسبعون، ينفع من البثور والقروح وخاصة في المفاصل. الخامس والسبعون، ينفع من أوجاع /35a/ المفاصل التي تكون من المواد الحارة. السادس والسبعون، يقلع البلغم اللزج الذي هو ملبس بجمل[104] المعدة ويحدره[105]. السابع والسبعون، يسهل المرة الصفراء إذا كثرت في المعدة وطال مقامها. الثامن والسبعون، ينفع من الجرب الحاد الأُكال. التاسع والسبعون، ينفع منفعة عجيبة من حدة الدم ويسكنها. الثمانون، يفتح السدد الحادثة في مجاري الطحال. الحادي والثمانون، ينفع أورام الكبد. الثاني والثمانون، ينفع الخفقان العارض في

الفؤاد. الثالث والثمانون، يحدر المرار الأسود المحتقن بالمعدة. الرابع والثمانون، ينفع من الجدري والحصبة. الخامس والثمانون، ينفع من قروح المثانة. السادس والثمانون، ينفع من سوء التنفس والإنتصاب. السابع والثمانون، يحدر[106] الطمث إذا تشوش الخدارة[107] في أوقاته. الثامن والثمانون، ينفع ميل الرحم إلى الجوانب.

السؤال الحادي عشر—كم حمد السكنجبين القليل الحموضة قوم؟

الجواب—من مسائل النجاد[108] حيث يقول: إنه إذا كان كذلك رطب الفم والحنك لتسكينه المرة الصفراء بما فيه من الحموضة وأعان على نفث النخامة[109] /35b/ وسكن العطش ووافق المواضع التي دون الشراسيف ومنع من حدوث المضار المعائية لأن طبع المعاء البرد واليبس ولأنها عصبية.

السؤال الثاني عشر—لم أمر أن يسقي السكنجبين في الأمراض الحادة قبل تناول ماء الشعير بساعتين وبعده بساعتين؟

الجواب—من مسائل النجاد، أما قبله فلأنه يجلو ويطفئ اللهب، وأما بعده فلأنه ينفذ ما يولده ماء الشعير.

السؤال الثالث عشر—ما هو القانون الكلي في مداواة حمى العفونة؟

الجواب—من الجزئيات لإبن سينا حيث يقول: الغرض في مداواة هذه الحميات تارة يتجه نحو الحمى فتحتاج أن تبرد وترطب وتارة نحو المادة حتى تحتاج أن تنضج أو[110] تستفرغ والإنضاج في الغليظ تعديله بالترقيق وفي الرقيق تعديله بالتغليظ وربما تناقض ما تستدعيه الحمى من التبريد والخلط من الإنضاج فحينئذ يجب أن يراعي الأهم من الأمرين فإن كانت القوّة قوية[111] قطعت السبب

ودبرت الخلط ومنعت[112] الغذاء[113] وإن كانت ضعيفة[114] إشتغلت بتعديل[115] المضاد[116] فبردته وأنعشت[117] القوّة بالغذاء[118].

السؤال الرابع عشر—ما هو القانون الكلي في معالجات أمراض العصب الخمسة أعني الخدر /36a/ والتشنج والرعشة والإختلاج والفالج؟

الجواب—من جزئيات القانون لإبن سينا، يقصد فيها فصد[119] مؤخر الدماغ ولا يعجل[120] بإستعمال الأدوية القوية بل يقتصر[121] على أشياء لطيفة مما يلين وينضج والحقن جيدة[122] ثم بآخره[123] يستعمل[124] المستفرغات القوية ويغذي[125] المفلوج في أول الأمر بماء العسل أو ماء الشعير[126] يومين أو[127] ثلاثة وإن إحتملت القوّة فإلى الرابع عشر وإجتهد في تجويعه و تعطيشه.

السؤال الخامس عشر—ما الفرق بين الدواء والغذاء؟

الجواب—من الأصول لإبن رضوان حيث يقول: الفرق من الغذاء والدواء أن الغذاء يتغير في البدن ويستحيل كيلوسه إلى أن يصير كيموساً من كيموسات البدن فمنه ما هو سريع التغير مثل الخمر ومنه ما هو وسط مثل الخبز ومنه ما هو بطيء مثل لحم البقر ومنه ما يغير البدن أولاً ثم يعود فيتغير عن يستحيل كيلوسه إلى بعض كيموسات البدن مثل الخس ويسمى ما كان كذلك غذاء دوائياً والدواء هو ما[128] غير البدن فمنه ما يغير البدن ثم يعود فيتغير عن[129] البدن وينقلب إليه ويسمى دواء غذائياً مثل الأدوية الحلوة ومنه ما يغير البدن وتضمحل[130] قوّته قليلاً قليلاً إما أن تدفعها طبيعة /36b/ البدن فتخرجه وإما أن ينقسم ويستحيل وتبطل قوّته ويسمى دواء على الإطلاق ومنه

عن البدن ما يغير البدن ولا يتغير عن البدن ويسمى ما كان كذلك دواء قتالاً.

السؤال السادس عشر—ما هو القانون الكلي في علاج القيء؟

الجواب—من الجزئيات لإبن سينا حيث يقول: ما كان من القيء متولداً عن فساد إستعمال الغذاء صلح[131] الغذاء وإستعين بمقويات المعدة الحارة العطرة[132] وما كان سببه مادة رديئة أو كثيرة إستفرغت تلك المادة على قوانين الإستفراغ[133] والحقن جيدة[134] والقيء أيضاً يقطع القيء إذا كان عن مادة، فإن كانت غليظة[136] بدأنا[137] فلطفناه ثم[138] قطعناه ثم إستفرغناه، وجذب المادة الهائجة إلى الأطراف نافع جدا في حبس[139] القيء، وإذا كانت الطبيعة يابسة فلا يحبس[140] القيء بما يجفف من القوابض إلا بقدر من غير إجحاف، وإذا قذف دواء مقوياً حابساً للقئ فأعده مرة أخرى[141] فإن[142] إشتدت كراهية[143] فغير[144] له شيئاً من رائحته أو لونه[145]، وإذا كان الغثيان على الخلو[146] فيحب أن يمتلئ[147] صاحبه وينقئ وأكثر الغثيان العارض عن حرارة ويبوسة يزول[148] بالتضميد المبرد المرطب[149] وأما الغثيان المادي فلا بد[150] من تنقيته[151] بما يليق ثم تعالج[152] الكيفية الباقية بما يضادها[153] من الأدوية العطرة مع الربوب حارة أو باردة لكل بحسبه.

السؤال السابع عشر—ما الفرق بين الضماد /37a/ والكماد؟

الجواب—من الأصول لإبن رضوان، إن الكماد يوضع وهو حار والضماد يوضع وهو بارد والقصد فيها أن يستفيد العضو قوّة أو تبديل مزاج حتى يعود إلى الإعتدال أو تحليل ما إجتمع فيه وإنضاجه أو دفعه إلى وراء أو منع ما يتحلب[154] أو ينصب أو يسخن[155] أجزاء العضو أو تقبيضها أو تليينها أو تصليبها

أو تلطيف ما حصل فيه أو تغليظه أو تقطيعه أو تلزيجه وتأليف الأدوية يكون بحسب المقصود إليه من هذه الأنحاء.

السؤال الثامن عشر—كم هي الأغراض المقصودة في حرق ما يحرق من الأدوية وغسل ما يغسل؟

الجواب—من كلام أمين الدولة إبن التلميذ حيث يقول: أما الأغراض المقصودة في حرق ما يحرق فخمسة، إما لتنقيص حدته كالقلقطار والزاج، وإما غسل ليكسب حدة كالنورة المحرقة، وإما لتلطيف كثافته[156] كالسرطان وقرن الأيل، وإما ليتهيأ للسحق كالإبريسم، وإما لأن تبطل رداءة جوهره[157]، وأما ما ينغسل فالأغراض المقصودة فيه ثلاثة، إزالة نارية مكتبسة كالنورة وإمكان التصويل كالتوتيا وإزالة قوّة مقصودة كقوّة التغشية[158] عن الحجر الأرمني.

السؤال التاسع عشر—ما هي الأمور الضارة بالمعدة والأمعاء؟

الجواب—من /37b/ جزئيات القانون، التخمة والإمتلاء ولذلك لا يخصب بدن النهم لأن طعامه لا ينهضم ولا يخصب[159] منه البدن، ومنع الريح والثفل عظيم الضرر فإنه ربما إرتد[160] الثفل من لفافة إلى لفافة إلى فوق[161] حتى يعود إلى المعدة فيؤذي أذاً[162] عظيماً، وكل ما لا قبض فيه من العصارات خاصة فهو رديء وجميع الأدهان ترخي[163] المعدة ولا توافقها[164] وأسلمها الزيت ودهن الفستق ومن الأدوية والأغذية الضارة بالمعدة في الأكثر حب الصنوبر والسلق والبادروج والسلجم غير[165] المهرأ بالطبخ والحماض والسرمق والبقلة اليمانية إلا بالخل والمري والزيت والحلبة والسمسم فإنهما يضعفان المعدة واللبن ضار للمعدة وكذلك[166] المخاخ

والأدمغة ومن الأشربة ما كان غليظاً ومن الأدوية حب العرعر وحب الفقد والأدوية المسهلة وجميع ما يستبشع[167] رديء للمعدة والجماع من أضر الأشياء بالمعدة[168] والقيء العنيف وإن نفع من جهة التنقية فهو يضر[169] ضرراً كثيراً[170] بالتضعيف[171].

السؤال العشرون—ما هي الأشياء الضارة بالكبد؟

الجواب—من جزئيات القانون[172] لإبن سينا[173] حيث يقول: إدخال طعام[174] على طعام[175] وإساءة ترتيبه من أضر الأشياء بالكبد وشرب[176] الماء البارد دفعة على الريق وفي إثر الحمام أو[177] الجماع أو[178] الرياضة /38a/ لأنه[179] ربما أدى إلى تبريد شديد[180] لحرص الكبد الملتهبة على الإمتياز[181] السريع[182] الكثير[183] منه ربما أدى إلى الإستسقاء ويجب في مثل هذه الحال أن يمزج ولايبرد تبريداً[184] شديداً ولا يعب عباً[185] بل يمص[186] قليلاً قليلاً مصاً[187] والأشياء اللزجة[188] كلها تضر بالكبد من جهة ما يؤرث السدد، والشراب الحلو يحدث في الكبد سدداً وهو في نفسه يجلو ما في الصدر.

الباب السابع فيما يسأل عنه الكحال وهو عشرون مسألة[1]

السؤال الأول—في أي أمراض العين يكتحل بعرق السوس؟

الجواب—من كلام[2] ديسقوريدوس مما نقله إبن وافد في أدويته المفردة حيث يقول: إن أصل السوس إذا قشر وسحق ونخل بمنخل صفيق وإكتحل به كان دواء نافعاً للظفرة في العين يذر عليها فيأكلها ويفنيها ويمحو أثرها ولذلك فعله باللحم الزائد الذي يخرج في[3] أصول الأظفار.

السؤال الثاني—كم هي الأسباب في رؤية الشئ الواحد إثنين؟

الجواب—من طبيعيات الشفاء لإبن سينا حيث يقول: إن السبب في رؤية الشئ[4] الواحد إثنين أربعة أسباب، أحدها إنفتال الآلة المؤدية للشبح الذي[5] في الجليدية إلى /38b/ ملتقي العصبتين فلا يتأدى الشبحان إلى موضع واحد على الإستقامة بل ينتهي كل عند جزء[6] من الروح الباصر المرتب[7] هناك على حدة لأن خطي الشبحين لم ينفذا نفوذاً من شأنه أن[8] يتقاطعا عند مجاورة ملتقي العصبتين فيجب لذلك أن ينطبع من كل شبح ينفذ عن الجليدية خيال على حدة وفي جزء[9] من الروح الباصر[10] على حدة فيكون كأنهما خيالان عن شيئين متفرقين من خارج إذ لم يتحد الخطان الخارجان منهما إلى مركز الجليدية[11] نافدين إلى[12] العصبتين. الثاني، حركة الروح الباصر[13] وتموجه يمنة ويسرة حتى يتقدم الجزء[14] المدرك مركزه[15] المرسوم له

في الطبع آخذاً إلى جهة الجليدية[16] أخذاً متموجاً مضطرباً فيرتسم فيه الشبح والخيال قبل تقاطع المخروطين فيرى شبحين وهذا مثل الشبح المرتسم من الشمس في الماء الراكد الساكن مرة واحدة والمرتسم منها في المتموج إرتساماً[17] متكرراً. الثالث، إضطراب حركة الروح الباطن الذي[18] وراء التقاطع إلى قدام وخلف حتى تكون لها حركتان إلى جهتين متضادتين حركة إلى الحس المشترك وحركة إلى ملتقي العصبتين فتتأدى إليهما[19] صورة المحسوس مرة قبل أن ينمحي ما تؤديه إلى الحس المشترك كأنها كما أدت الصورة إلى الحس المشترك رجع منها جزء يقبل ما تؤديه القوّة الباصرة /39a/ وذلك بسرعة الحركة فيكون مثلاً قد إرتسم في الروح المؤدية صورة فتقبلها[20] إلى الحس المشترك ولكل مرتسم زمان ثبات إلى أن ينمحي فلما[21] زال القابل الأول من الروح عن مركزه لإضطراب حركته خلفه جزء آخر فقبل قبوله قبل أن إنمحى[22] عن الأول فتحركت[23] الروح للإضطراب إلى جزء متقدم كان[24] في سمت المرئي فأدركه ثم زال ولم تزل عنه الصورة دفعة بل هي فيه وإلى جزء آخر[25] قابل للصورة أيضاً بحصوله في السمت الذي في مثله يدرك[26] الصورة عاقباً للجزء الأول والسبب الإضطراب. الرابع، إضطراب حركة تعرض للثقبة العينية فإن الطبقة العينية[27] سهلة[28] الحركة إلى هيئة تتسع لها الثقبة وتضيق تارة إلى خارج وتارة إلى داخل على الإستقامة أو إلى جهة فيتبع إندفاعها إلى [خارج إنضغاط يعرض لها وإتساع من الثقبة ويتبع إندفاعها إلى][29] داخل إجتماع يعرض لها فإذا إتفق أن ضاقت الثقبة ترى أكبر أو إتسعت ترى الشئ أصغر و[30] إتفق أن مالت إلى جهة رأى[31] في مكان آخر فيكون كأن المرئي أولاً غير المرئي ثانياً وخصوصاً

إذا كان قد تمثل قبل إنمحاء الصورة الأولى صورة أخرى.

السؤال الثالث—في أي أمراض العين يذر بالقصب البالي العتيق[32] فيبرأ؟

الجواب—من الملكي حيث يقول: إن القصب البالي العتيق إذا سحق ناعماً[33] وذر به /39b/ العين نفع[34] البياض.

السؤال الرابع—كم هي الأمور الضارة بالنظر وما هي؟

الجواب—من الكتاب الثالث من القانون حيث يقول: إنها ثلاثة، أحدها أفعال وحركات. الثاني أغذية. الثالث حال التصرف في الأغذية. أما[35] الأفعال[36] فمثل[37] الجماع الكثير وطول النظر في المضيئات وقراءة الدقيق قراءة تأمل[38] بإفراط فإن التوسط فيها نافع وكذلك الأعمال الدقيقة والنوم على الإمتلاء والعشاء بل يجب على من به ضعف في البصر أن يصبر حتى ينهضم ثم ينام وكل امتلاء يضره[39] وكل ما يجفف الطبيعة يضر[40] أيضاً[41] وكل ما يعكر الدم من الأشياء المالحة والحريفة والسكر. وأما القئ فينفعه من حيث أنه[42] ينقي المعدة ويضره من حيث أنه[43] يحرك مواد الدماغ فيدفعها إليه وإن كان لا بد فينبغي أن يكون بعد الطعام ويرفق والإستحمام ضار والنوم المفرط ضار والبكاء الكثير ضار[44] وكثرة الفصد وخصوصاً الحجامة المتوالية ضارة. وأما الأغذية الضارة[45] فالمنخرة[46] والمالحة والحريفة وما يؤذي فم المعدة والكراث والبصل والثوم والبادروج أكلاً والزيتون والكرنب والشبث[47] والعدس. وأما التصرف في الأغذية فإن يتناولها ويحترز من فسادها[48] وكثرة بخارها.

السؤال الخامس—إذا رأيت العين كحلاء كيف /40a/ تعلم أنها من قبل

الطبقات؟

الجواب—من القانون، أما الكحلاء بسبب الرطوبات فيكون بصرها بالليل أقل بسبب أن ذلك يحتاج إلى تحديق وتحريك للمادة إلى خارج والمادة الكثيرة تكون أعصى[49] من القليل وأما الكحلاء بسبب الطبقات[50] فيجمع البصر أشد.

السؤال السادس—كيف يعلم أن العين الزرقاء بسبب قلة الرطوبة البيضية وما علة ذلك؟

الجواب—هذه تكون[51] أبصر بالليل وفي الظلمة[52] من النهار[53] لما يعرض من تحريك الضوء للمادة القليلة فيشغلها عن التبين[54] فإن مثل[55] هذه الحركة تعجز[56] عن تبيين الأشياء كما تعجز[57] عن تبين ما في الظلمة.

السؤال السابع—ما هي القوانين الكلّيّة في معالجات أمراض العين؟

الجواب—لما كانت الأمراض إما مزاجية مادية وإما مزاجية ساذجة وإما تركيبية وإما[58] تفرق إتصال[59] فعلاج العين إما إسستفراغ فيدخل فيه تدبير الأورام وإما تبديل مزاج وإما إصلاح هيئة كما في الجحوظ وإما إدمال وإلحام والعين تستفرغ المواد عنها إما على سبيل الصرف عنها وإما على سبيل التجليب منها والمصرف[60] عنها هو أولى من البدن إن كان ممتلئاً وأما التجليب منها فيكون[61] بالأدوية المدمعة[62] وأما تبديل المزاج فيقع بأدوية خاصية وأما تفرق الإتصال فيعالج بالأدوية التي تجفف يسيراً وهي[63] بعيدة من اللذع.

السؤال الثامن—/40b/ إذا كان مع وجع العين صداع شديد فأيهما[64]

يبدأ يعالجه[65]؟

الجواب—يبدأ[66] في العلاج بالصداع ولا يعالج[67] العين قبل أن يزيله[68] وإذا لم يعن[69] الإستفراغ والتنقية والتدبير الجيد[70] فإعلم أن في العين مزاجاً رديئاً أو مادة رديئة تحجب[71] في الطبقات تفسد الغذاء الوارد[72] إليها أو هناك ضعف في الدماغ أو[73] في موضع تنقذف منه النوازل إلى العين.

السؤال التاسع—ما هو[74] من أجزاء العين إذا[75] مرض مرضاً مخصوصاً أنقعت[76] العين بذلك ولم تبصر[77]؟

الجواب—من المقالة الثالثة من التذكرة حيث يقول: إذا تشنج[78] العضل المثلث الذي على فم العصبة النورية فأنها تشد العين وتربطها.

السؤال العاشر—كم هي أسباب الشبكرة؟

الجواب—خمسة[79] أسباب، من المقالة الثالثة من التذكرة، إما من رطوبة تعرض للبيضية وإما لغلظ[80] الروح النفساني وإما لرطوبة[81] الجليدية وكدورتها وإما من مداواة الشمس وإما من قبل بخار من المعدة.

السؤال الحادي عشر—كم هي أمراض البيضية؟

الجواب—سبعة، تغير لونها جفوفها[82] جوف جزء منها صغرها كبرها رطوبتها غلظها.

السؤال الثاني عشر—على كم وجه يكون[83] /41a/ تغير البيضية في اللون؟

الجواب—ثلاثة، أما إن تتغير كلها فيرى الجسم كله باللون الذي هو[84] عليه.

الثاني أنه ربما تغيرت في بعض الأوقات بسبب بخارات تتصاعد[84] إليها من المعدة فترى[86] الأجسام على حسب ذلك البخار. الثالث أنه إن كان قد[87] تغير بعض أجزائها فيرى من أصابه بين يديه أجساماً شبيهة في ألوانها وأشكالها بأجزاء تلك الرطوبة.

السؤال الثالث عشر—كم هي الأمراض الخاصية بالأجفان؟

الجواب—إثنا عشر—الجرب، والبرد، والتحجر، والإلتصاق، والشترة، والشعيرة، والشعر الزائد، وإنقلاب الشعر، والوردينج، والسلاق، والشرناق.

السؤال الرابع عشر—من كم سبب يكون مرض من يبصر[88] بالليل ولايبصر[89] بالنهار؟

الجواب—ثلاثة، إما من شدة يبس الروح الحيواني[90] النوري وإما من[91] قلته وضعفه وإما من إفراط التحليل[92].

السؤال الخامس عشر—ما الفرق بين الإتساع والإنتشار؟

الجواب—من التذكرة، إن[93] الإتساع يحدث في الطبقة أو العصبة والإنتشار في النور فالإتساع مرض والإنتشار عرض.

السؤال السادس عشر—كم هي الأشياء التي لأجلها إستعملت الأشياء الرطبة اللزجة في العين؟

الجواب—من التذكرة، أربعة، أحدها أنها[94] غير لذاعة /41b/. الثاني لتغرى[95] الخشونة الكائنة عن الحدة وتغسلها. الثالث أنها تبقى في العين أكثر من بقاء الرطوبة المائية. الرابع أن العين عضو له حس[96] وأكثر الأدوية التي تعالج بها حجرية[97] وكل شئ خشن إذا لقي[98] كثير الحس آذاه إختار[99] الأطباء أن يخلطوا في

أدويتها شيئاً يلين خشونتها وهي لطيفة كبياض[100] البيض وماء الحلبة وماء الصمغ والكثيراء ونحوها[101].

السؤال السابع عشر—ما الفرق بين الجساء العارض للجفن وبين الغلظ؟

الجواب—من التذكرة، إن الجساء لا يكون[102] معه نفخة وهو صلابة تعرض للجفن ويعرض ذلك في جفن واحد أو فيهما وسببه برد ويبس[103] والغلظ[104] معه نفخة ويكون[105] في الجفنين جميعاً وسببه مادة باردة رطبة غليظة[106].

السؤال الثامن عشر—ما الفرق بين نتوء العنبية وبين البثر الحادث في القرنية؟

الجواب—من التذكرة، ينبغي أن تنظر إلى لون العنبية ما هو ثم تقيس[107] لون ذلك إلى العلة فإن لم يكن على لونها علمت [أنها بثرة وتنظر أيضاً إلى نفس الحدقة فإن كانت قد صغرت أو أعوجت عن إستدارتها علمت][108] أنه نتوء في القرنية وإن لم ترشيئاً مما ذكرت فهي بثرة فإن كان[109] على لون العنبية فأنظر إلى أصل الشئ الناتئ وإلى نفس[110] الحدقة فإن رأيت أصل الشئ الناتئ أثر بياض فإعلم أن ذلك الشئ الأبيض خرق القرنية والشئ الناتئ من العنبية وإن لم تر شيئاً من ذلك فهي بثرة. /42a/

السؤال التاسع عشر—بماذا يفرق بين نتوء القرنية والبثر الحادث فيها؟

الجواب—أما نتوءها فصلب جاس[111] وإذا غمزت عليه بالميل لم ينخفض لصلابته وأما البثر فتتبعها دمعة وضربان ويكون لونها أحمر إلى البياض.

السؤال العشرون—في أي زمان من أزمنة المرض تستعمل الذرورات؟

الجواب—من التذكرة، إياك أن تستعمل الذرورات في الإبتداء لا في الرمد ولا في القروح لأن آفته عظيمة الا[112] إن كنت على ثقة من نقاء البدن والرأس ثم قال: وإحذر أن تستعمل في الإبتداء والصعود ذروراً فيه أنزروت فأنه يجلب على المريض أذية عظيمة[113].

الباب الثامن فيما يسأل عنه الجرائحي وهو عشرون مسألة[1]

السؤال الأول—كم هي العظام التي في البدن؟

الجواب—من القانون وقد حرره إبن جميع وهي على ما يأتي[2] تفصيله مائتان وستة وأربعون عظماً تفصيله القحف إثنان، وما دون القحف خمسة، الزوج أربعة، اللحي الأعلى إثناعشر، الأنف إثنان، الأسنان إثنان وثلاثون، اللحي الأسفل إثنان، فقرات /42b/ الصلب ثلاثون، الأضلاع أربعة وعشرون، القص سبعة، الكتفان إثنان، الترقوتان إثنان، العضدان إثنان، الساعدان أربعة، الرسفان ستة عشر، المشطان ثمانية، الأصابع ثلاثون، العانة إثنان، الفخذان إثنان، الساقان أربعة، القدمان إثنان وخمسون، هذا كلام إبن جميع. وأما صاحب القانون فيقول: إنها مائتان و ثمانية وأربعون[3] عظماً سوى السمسمانية والشبيه باللام[4]. قال إبن جميع: و العظمان الباقيان هما رأسا الكتفين.

السؤال الثاني—كم هي عضل البدن؟

الجواب—خمسمائة تسعة وعشرون عضلة، تفصيل ذلك الوجه تسعة، العينان[5] أربعة وعشرون، اللحي الأسفل إثناعشر، الفكان[6] أربعة عشر، الرأس ثلاثة وعشرون، قصبة الرئة أربعة، الحنجرة ستة عشر، العظم الشبيه باللام ستة، اللسان تسعة، الحلق إثنان، الرقبة أربعة، مفصل الكتفين مع العضدين ستة

وعشرون، المرفقان[7] ثمانية، الساعدان[8] أربعة وثلاثون، الكفان[9] ستة وثلاثون، الصدر مائة وسبعة، الصلب ثمانية وأربعون، البطن ثمانية، المثانة واحدة، القضيب أربعة، الأُنثيان[10] أربعة، الشرج أربعة، وعلى الوركين لحركة[11] الفخذين ستة وعشرون، وعلى الفخذين لحركة[12] الساقين عشرون، وعلى الساقين ثمانية وعشرون، وعلى القدمين إثنان وخمسون، وقيل خمسة وخمسون /43a/.

السؤال الثالث—كم هي أعصاب البدن الدماغية النخاعية وغيرها[13]؟

الجواب—ثمان وثلاثون زوجاً وفرد لا أخ له، تفصيل ذلك الدماغية سبعة، النخاعية أحد وثلاثون زوجاً[14]، وفرد لا أخ له منها من فقار العنق ثمانية أزواج ومنها من فقار الصدر إثناعشر زوجاً ومنها من فقار القطن خمسة[15] أزواج ومنها من عظام العجر ثلاثة أزواج ومن طرف عظم العصعص الأخير يخرج عصب فرد لا أخ له.

السؤال الرابع—كم عدد العروق التي تفصد في الأكثر؟

الجواب—ثلاثة وثلاثون عرقاً منها إثنا[16] عشر في اليدين قيفالان وباسليقان إنسيان[17] وباسليقان إبطيان[18] والكحلان[19] وحبلا الذراع وأسيلمان ومنها في الرأس والرقبة ثلاثة عشر عرقا الصدغان[20] وعرقان خلف الأُذنين وعرقا المأقين وعرقا الوداجين وعرق[21] اليافوخ وعرق الجبهة وعرق مؤخر الرأس وعرق الأرنبة وعرق تحت اللسان هذا قول صاحب الملكي ورأيت في هذا الموضع حاشية ثم الجهارك الأربعة إثنان في الشفة[22] العليا وإثنان في الشفة السفلى وفي الرجلين ثمان عروق عرقان في مابض[23] الركبتين وعرقا الساقين وعرقا النساء وعرقا مشطي

القدمين.

السؤال الخامس—كم هي الأصول التي /43b/ يجب أن ينظر فيها عند مداواة تفرق الإتصال الواقع في الأعضاء اللينة؟

الجواب—من الكلّيّات، الغرض من علاجة أمور ثلاثة، الأول[24] إن كان لسبب ثابتاً فأول ما يجب هو[25] قطع ما يسيل وقطع مادته إن كانت حافزة[26]، الثاني الحام الشق بالأدوية والأغذية الموافقة، والثالث منع العفونة ما أمكن.

السؤال السادس—كم هي الأشياء المانعة من برء القرحة وكيف يتدارك كل واحد منها؟

الجواب—من الكلّيّات، أربعة، مزاج العضو ويجب أن يعني[27] بإصلاحه، الثاني رداءة مزاج الدم المتوجه إليه ويجب أن يتدارك[28] بما يولد الكيموس المحمود، الثالث كثرة الدم الذي يسيل إليه ويتدارك[29] بالإستفراغ وتلطيف الغذاء وإستعمال الرياضة إن أمكن، الرابع فساد العظم الذي تحته وارسالة الصديد[30] وهذا لا دواء له إلا إصلاح ذلك العظم وحكه إن كان الحك يأتي على فساده أو أخذه وقطعه.

السؤال السابع—أي الأدوية التي ينبغي عملها في قروح الإحليل؟

الجواب—من المقالة الرابعة من حيلة البرء لجالينوس حيث يقول: قروح الإحليل تحتاج إلى كثرة التجفيف بحسب فضل يبسه في طبعه بمنزلة القرطاس المحرق والشب المحرق والقرع اليابس المحرق والصبر في أول الأمر يستحق أيها كان /44a/ أو ما يجري مجراها وينثر على القرحة.

السؤال الثامن—كيف تكون الحال إذا أصابت العصبة نخسة وكيف يكون طريق مداواتها؟

الجواب—من المقالة السادسة من كتاب حيلة البرء لجالينوس حيث يقول: إذا أصابت عصبة نخسة فلا بد ضرورة لفضل حسه من أن يناله وجع شديد أكثر من سائر الأعضاء ولذلك لا محالة له يرم إن لم يحتل له في تسكين الوجع ومنع حدوث الورم وذلك يكون[31] بأن يستبقى موضع الخرق من الجلد على حاله ويمنع من الإلتحام ليخرج ما يرشح من موضع النخسة من الصديد ينقى البدن كله من الفضول بفصد العرق إن كان ثم قوّة تحتمل وتنقية الأخلاط الرديئة بدواء مسهل تبادر به في أول الأمر وإن توسع الجرح وينطل بالزيت الذي لا قبض[32] فيه بعد أن يسخن والأجود إن يكون الزيت الذي قد أتت عليه سنتان أو ثلاثة فإن هذا يحلل أكثر ويختار من الأدوية ما كان لطيف الأجزاء معتدل الحرارة يجفف بلا أذى معه مثل علك البطم واليسير من الفربيون ووسخ الكور والسكبينج والجاوشير والحلتيت[33] في الأبدان الصلبة والكبريت الذي لم يصبه نار يخلط أي هذه كان بالزيت حتى يصير في ثخن العسل ويضمد به الجرح.

السؤال التاسع—هل يجوز أن يستعمل في قروح /44b/ العصب شيئاً من الأشياء المرخية أو يستعمل الماء الحار؟

الجواب—من المقالة السادسة من حيلة البرء حيث يقول: وإياك أن تستعمل في قروح العصب الماء الحار والأشياء من الأدوية المرخية.

السؤال العاشر—كم هي الخصال التي يحتاج إليها في جراحات المراق؟

الجواب—من المقالة السادسة من حيلة البرء لجالينوس وهي أربع خصال وذلك حيث يقول: وجراحات المراق تحتاج إلى أربع خصال أحدها أن يخيط الجراحة، الثاني أن يدخل ما يخرج أو يبرز من الأمعاء إلى موضعه، الثالث وضع الدواء الموافق، الرابع أن لا تدع غاية في الحرص على أن لا يلحق شيئاً من الأعضاء الشريفة آفة بسبب الجراحة.

السؤال الحادي عشر—إذا برز المعاء وبرده الهواء فإنتفخ، كيف يداوي؟

الجواب—من المقالة السادسة من حيلة البرء حيث يقول: يحتاج إلى الإسخان لينحل الريح منه وإسخانه بإسفنجة تغمس في ماء حار وتعصر ويكمد بها والشراب القابض إذا سخن نفع من ذلك وجمع مع إسخانه تقوية الأمعاء فإن بقي على حاله في الإنتفاخ وكان الجرح ضيقاً فينبغي أن يشق الصفاق بمقدار ما يحتاج إليه المعاء البارز في دخوله.

السؤال /45a/ **الثاني عشر**—القروح التي في عرض العضلة هل الطريق في مداواتها هو مثل القروح الحادثة في طولها؟

الجواب—من حيلة البرء لجالينوس حيث يقول: القروح الذاهبة في عرض العضلة شقيها[34] أشد تباعداً فيحتاج أن تجمع شقيها[35] جمعاً أشد وأبلغ ولذلك يحتاج الخياطة <u>ويرفدها بعد الخياطة</u>[36] برفائد مثلثة والقروح الذاهبة في طول العضلة يلتقي بالرباط اللهم إلا أن تكون الجراحة مفرطة فيحتاج إلى خياطة يسيرة أو رفائد بلا خياطة.

السؤال الثالث عشر—كم هي منافع الفصد؟

الجواب—من كتاب الفصد لجالينوس ضربان، أحدهما إزالة الإمتلاء والآخر إبطال المرض الذي يتوقع حدوثه عن ضربة أو ألم شديد أو عن ضعف العضو وقبوله لما يدفع إليه الأعضاء.

السؤال الرابع عشر—كيف طريق مداواة الجراحة إذا وقعت بالرأس وبلغت إلى نواحي الغشاء؟

الجواب—من الملكي من المقالة الرابعة عشر منه[37] حيث يقول: متى وقعت بالرأس جراحة وبلغت إلى نواحي الدماغ والغشاء فلا ينبغي أن يبادر بالأدوية[38] التي تدمل وتلحم فإنك إن فعلت ذلك جلبت على العليل العطب لأنه يرم[39] الدماغ /45b/ ويختلط[40] العقل ويحدث التشنج لكن تجعل فيها[41] صوفة قد غمست في زيت ثلاثة أيام لتأمن[42] الورم والتشنج ثم من[43] بعد ذلك تستعمل[44] المراهم والذرورات الملحمة بمنزلة الذرور المعمول من المر والصبر والكندر والمرهم الأسود وما يشاكل[45] ذلك[46].

السؤال الخامس عشر—كيف طريق مداواة القرحة مع عظم مكسور؟

الجواب—من المقالة الرابعة عشر من الملكي حيث يقول: متى تركبت القرحة مع عظم مكسور فعالج[47] العظم مع ما يعالج[48] القرحة بالضماد القوي[49] الذي[50] يستعمل في جبر العظام المكسورة فإن وقعت الجراحة بالرأس وإنكسر عظم القحف ولم يضر بالغشاء فينبغي أن يضمد[51] العظم بالزراوند المدحرج مدقوقاً ناعماً معجوناً بالماء فإنه يخرج العظم ثم يعالج بعد ذلك بالمر والكندس[52] أجزاء سواء[53] مدقوقاً منخولاً معجوناً بالعسل وشراب مطبوخ حتى ينعقد والطخه على[54] فتيلة

وإستعمله بالمراهم.

السؤال السادس عشر—كيف طريق مداواة القروح إذا كان تحتها عظم قد عفن وما علامة ذلك؟

الجواب—من الملكي أما علامته فإن ترى[55] القرحة تندمل إحياناً ثم تعود فتنفتح ويسيل منها صديد وإذا أدخلت رأس المجس في القرحة أحسست له بخشخشة فإذا علمت[56] ذلك فإلزمه /46a/ المرهم[57] الحاد ليأكل اللحم الميت فإذا فعلت ذلك وصار الموضع كالخشكريشة أو كاللحم الرخو[58] فالسمن[59] المفتر حتى يسقط اللحم المحترق[60] وينكشف العظم فإذا بان[61] لك العظم وأمكن قطعه فإقطعه وإلا فالسمن[62] المفتر ثانية حتى تعفن[63] ويسقط ثم يعالج يوماً بمرهم الزنجار و يوماً بالقطن الخلق حتى ينبت اللحم ويندمل.

السؤال السابع عشر—بماذا يخرج الشوك والأزجة إذا دخلت في بعض الأعضاء وصارت إلى موضع لا يمكن إخراجه بالحديد؟

الجواب—من الملكي، ينبغي أن يوضع على الموضع الذي دخلت فيه الزراوند المدحرج مدقوقاً ناعماً معجوناً بالاُشق يلزم ذلك أياماً أو يؤخذ أصول القصب الفارسي الرطب فيدق ناعما[64] ويخلط بالعسل ويلزم الموضع أو يؤخذ علك الأنباط وزفت يذوبان ويخلط معهما أذان الفار مسحوقاً ناعماً فإنه يجذبه ويخرجه.

السؤال الثامن عشر—كيف يسمى تفرق الإتصال الحادث في عضو[65]؟

الجواب—من الكلّيّات، إن وقع في الجلد سمي سحجاً و خدشاً[66] وإن وقع

في اللحم ولم يقح[67] سمي جراحة وإن قيح[68] سمي قرحة وإن وقع في العظم سمي كسراً وإن وقع في طوله كان[69] صدعاً وإن وقع في عرض العصب سمي بتراً وإن وقع /46b/ طولاً ولم يكن كثير العدد[70] سمي شقاً وإن كان عدده كثيراً[71] سمي شدخاً وإن وقع في[72] طرف العضلة سمي هتكاً سواء كان في عصبة أو في وتر وإن وقع في عرض العضلة سمي جزاً وإن وقع في الطول وكثر غوره وقل عدده[73] سمي فدغاً وإن كثرت أجزاءه وفشا وغار سمي رضاً فسخاً وربما قيل الفسخ والرض والفدغ لكل ما يتفق في وسط العضلة كيف كان وإن وقع في الشرايين سمي أم الدم[74] وإن وقع في الأوردة سمي إنفجاراً وإن إعترضها[75] سمي قطعاً وفصلاً وإن نفذ[76] في طولها سمي صدعاً وإن إنفتحت[77] فوهاتها سمي ثيقاً[78] وإن كان في الأغشية والحجب سمي فتقاً وإن وقع بين جزئين من عضو مركب ففصل[79] أحدهما عن[80] الآخرمن غير أن ينال العضو المتشابه الأجزاء تفرق إتصال سمي إنفصالاً وخلعاً وإن كان في عصب زال عن موضعه سمي فكاً.

السؤال التاسع عشر—كم هي الفصول التي ينبغي لمن يطهر أن ينظر فيها قبل التطهير و بعده؟

الجواب—من[81] رسالة أحمد بن علي الفارسي في التطهير حيث يقول: ينبغي أن ينظر في سبعة فصول، الأول ينبغي[82] أن ينقى البدن قبل التطهير، الثاني في الأغذية التي تصلح لمن تطهر، الثالث في كيفية القطع والآلة التي /47a/ يكون بها القطع، الرابع في الذرورات التي تقطع الدم، الخامس في المراهم التي تصلح له خاصة، السادس في المراهم التي تغسل الإحليل، السابع في دخول الحمام والوقت

الذي يجب فيه.

السؤال العشرون—ما هو المرهم المخصوص بالإحليل[83] عند التطهير وفي أي وقت يعمل؟

الجواب—من رسالة السوسي في التطهير، قال: مرهم بديع التركيب يصلح لأبدان الصبيان والأبدان الرطبة ويعمل في الويم الثاني من التطهير صفته دهن ورد نصف رطل مرداسنج ربع رطل[84] يدق وينخل حتى يصير مثل الكحل ويطبخ مع الدهن حتى يصير كالشمع لا يلطخ اليد وينزل عن النار ويلقى عليه عشرة[85] دراهم شمع مقصور أبيض[86] وأوقية سمن بقري وعشرة دراهم أقاقيا محرقة مغسولة بماء الورد مدقوقة منخولة وسبعة دراهم صبر أسقطري ويطبخ بنار لينة ويحرك دائماً حتى يصير كالشمع ويرفع.

الباب التاسع فيما يسأل عنه المجبر[1] وهو عشرون مسئلة

السؤال الأول—ما هو العضو الصعب الإنخلاع والعضو السهل الإنخلاع والمتوسط؟

الجواب—من /47b/ الكتاب الرابع من القانون حيث يقول: السهلة الإنخلاع مثل مفصل الركبة لسلاسة رباطه وهو سهل الإرتداد[2] أيضاً[3] ومفصل المنكب قريب من ذلك[4] في المهازيل والصعبة الإنخلاع مثل مفاصل[5] الأصابع فإنها لا تكاد[6] تنخلع بل تنكسر قبل أن تنخلع ومثل مفصل المرفق ولذلك ردها صعب وأما المتوسط فمثل مفصل الورك فأصعب الخلع ما تنقطع[7] معه رؤوس شظايا العظم[8] الذي يلزق عظماً بعظم وقلما يرجع إلى حاله الطبيعية وأكثر ذلك في رأس الورك ثم في رأس العضد وفي زندي القدمين عند الكسر.

السؤال الثاني—ما هي علامات الخلع وما هي علامات الميل وما هي علامات طول المفصل من غير خلع؟

الجواب—الخلع يحدث في المفصل إنخفاض وغؤور[9] غير معهود مثل ما يعرض في مفصل الرجل وأظهر من[10] ذلك في مفصل العنق والمقائسة مما يخرج ذلك إخراجاً صحيحاً وهو أن تعتبر العليلة بأختها الصحيحة وإذا رأيت المفصل لا يتحرك حركته إلى جميع جهاته فليس به علة متعلقة بالزوال وأما علامات الميل فهو

أن يرى[11] تقعيراً مع نتوء في[12] جانب آخر مع أن بعض الحركة ممكنة[13] وأما علامات زيادة طول المفصل من غير /48a/ خلع فهو أن يكون كالمتعلق فإذا إدغمته إرتد إلى موضعه[14] الطبيعي من غير تكلف وإن تركته عاد إلى القد[15] العرضي وحدث غؤور وربما دخل[16] فيه[17] الإصبع حيث لا يكون اللحم شديد الكثرة مثل المنكب.

السؤال الثالث—كم هي أنواع كسر القحف البسيط؟

الجواب—من الملكي، ستة حيث يقول: إن الكسر الذي يعرض للقحف منه بسيط ومنه مركب والبسيط منه ما هو في الرأس[18] ظاهراً له عمق إلا أنه لم ينفصل فيه العظم ولا زال عنه[19] جزء لا إلى خارج ولا إلى داخل ومنه شق يكون[20] مع خروج العظم المكسور ومنه ما ينكسر[21] القحف بأجزاء كثيرة ويكون كسر العظام قد صارت[22] إلى العمق فيما[23] يلي الأم الجافية ومنه ما يصير العظم المكسور إلى أسفل قريباً من الصفاق ومنه شق عظيم[24] الرأس ومصيره مع دخول العظم إلى داخل ومنه النوع الشعري وهو شق دقيق يخفى عن الحس[25] فلا يتبين وربما كان سبباً للهلاك.

السؤال الرابع—ما هو الهشم وعلى كم وجه يكون؟

الجواب—من الملكي، حيث يقول: وأما الهشم فليس هو شق العظم[26] ولكنه عطف العظم إلى داخل وتعقده[27] من غير أن ينفصل إتصاله كالذي يعرض لآنية الرصاص والفضة /48b/ إذا صدمها[28] جرم أصلب منها[29] وهو على وجهين وذلك أنه إما أن ينهشم سمكه[30] كله حتى أنه كثيراً ما يدفع أم الدماغ وإما أن يصعد[31] عظم الرأس لسطح الأم التي[32] على القحف.

السؤال الخامس—أيما أسرع علاجاً وأسهل العظم المكسور المتبرئ أو

العظم المكسور غير المتبرئ؟

الجواب—من الملكي، المتبرئ أسهل وذلك لأن المتبرئ يمكن[33] فيه المد والتسوية ورده إلى شكله وغير المتبرئ لا يمكن فيه ذلك[34].

السؤال السادس—أيما[35] أسرع برءًا[36] في كسر الذراع كسر القصبة الغليظة أو[37] الدقيقة أو كسرهما؟

الجواب—من الملكي، أما كسرهما معاً فأصعب علاجاً وأشد نكاية[38] ولاسيما إن إنكسرا في موضع واحد[39] وأما كسر الغليظة[40] فهو أبطأ برءًا[41] وأردأ وأما كسر الأدق فهو أسرع برءًا.

السؤال السابع—ما هو الخلع وما هو زوال المفصل؟

الجواب—من الملكي، إن الخلع هو خروج زائدة العظم من حفرته المركبة فيها فإن كان الخروج يسيراً ولم يبرز[42] من الحفرة لم يقال له[43] خلع لكن يقال له زوال المفصل.

السؤال الثامن—ما الذي يعرض من إنخلاع عظمي الفك إذا تركا وأهملا؟

الجواب—قال /49a/ صاحب الملكي: فإنه إن تركا ولم يردا حدث عن ذلك أعراض رديئة منها حميات دائمة وصداع دائم وذلك أن عضل[44] الفكين إذا تغير عن موضعه تمدد[45] وجذب معه عضل[46] الصدغين ومددهما وعرض[47] من ذلك الصداع الشديد ويحدث لصاحب هذه الحال إسهال وقيء مرتين[48] صرفتين[49] وكثيراً ما يموت في العاشر.

السؤال التاسع—كم هي الوجوه الأكثرية التي يخرج مفصل الورك إليها؟

الجواب—من الملكي، أربعة أحدها أن ينتقل عن موضعه إلى داخل، الثاني أن ينتقل من موضعه[50] إلى خارج[51]، الثالث أن ينتقل[52] إلى قدام، الرابع إلى خلف وإنتقاله إلى قدام أقل ما يكون وإلى داخل أكثر ما يكون.

السؤال العاشر—كم هي أوجه الخلع التي تعرض لمفصل الركبة؟

الجواب—من الملكي، ثلاثة أحدها أن ينخلع إلى داخل، والثاني إلى خارج، الثالث إلى خلف و ليس ينخلع إلى قدام لأن فلكة الركبة تمنعه من ذلك.

السؤال الحادي عشر—ما الذي يجب على المجبر يتأمله؟

الجواب—من القانون، قال: ويجب على المجبر أن يتأمل ميل العظم المكسور فإنه يجد عند الجهة التي الميل[53] إليها حدبة وعند الجهة المميل عنها /49b/ تقعيراً وأكثر ما يفطن[54] لذلك باللمس وأيضاً فإن الوجع يشتد في الجهة التي إليها الميل ويجب عليه[55] أن يمر يده على موضع الكسر في كل حال أمراراً إلى فوق وإلى أسفل بالرفق ولا يجب أن يغير بالإستواء المحسوس بالبصر قبل تمام العافية فإن الورم قد يخفى كثيراً من الإعوجاج ويجب أن يبادر[56] إلى جبر ما إنكسر فيجبره في يومه فإنه كلما طال كان إدخاله أعسر والآفات فيه أكثر وخصوصاً العظام التي يحيط[57] بها عضل.

السؤال الثاني عشر—ما هو الوقت الذي تستعمل فيه الجبائر؟

الجواب—من القانون، هو بعد خمسة أيام وما[58] فوقها إلى أن تؤمن الآفات

وكلما عظم العضو وجب أن يبطأ[59] بوضع الجبائر وكثيراً ما يجلب الإستعجال في ذلك آفات[60] لكن يجعل ما يقوم مقامها من جودة الرباط[61] بالعصائب وجودة[62] النصبة[63] فإن لم يمكن ذلك فلا بد من الجبائر ولو في أول الأمر ويجب أن تلزم الجبائر الرباطات إلزاماً محكماً[64] ويكون[65] عند الكسر ويجب للضرورة أن تحل الرباطات[66] في كل يومين في أول الأمر وخصوصاً إن[67] حدثت حكة فإذا مضى[68] السابع من الشد فيحل[69] في كل أربعة أيام أو[70] خمسة ويرخى قليلاً من الرباط فإن أمكنك إبقاء الجبائر ولو عشرين يوماً ولم يمكن مضرة[71] فلا تحلها /50a/.

السؤال الثالث عشر—ما قاعدة الجبر؟

الجواب—من القانون، الجبر قاعدته مد العضو بمقدار ما ينبغي فإن الزيادة فيه تشنج و تؤلم وتحدث فيه[72] حميات وربما عرض منه إسترخاء وذلك في الأبدان الرطبة أقل ضرراً لمؤاتاتها للمد والنقصان منه يمنع جودة الإلتئام والنظم وهذا في الخلع والكسر سواء ويجب أن يسكن العضو ما أمكن إلا إحياناً بقدر ما يحتمل إذا لم تكن آفة أو[73] ورم لئلا تموت[74] طبيعة العضو ويجب أن يحذر الإيجاع الشديد عند المد والشد في الكسر والخلع معاً.

السؤال الرابع عشر—ما من العظام لا ينبت عليها دشبد[75]؟

الجواب—من القانون في الكتاب الرابع[76] في ذكر أصول الجبر والربط،

قال: المراد في أكثر الجبر حدوث الدشبد فيما ليس لعظام[77] الرأس فإنها لا ينبت عليها دشبد.

السؤال الخامس عشر—كيف يكون الشد إذا كان الكسر بالطول وهل هو

مثل الشد إذا كان الكسر بالعرض أم لا؟

الجواب—من الكتاب الرابع من القانون حيث يقول: وأما الكسر بالطول فيكتفي[78] فيه أن يلزم العضو بشد شديد أشد مما في غيره ويبالغ[79] في غمزه إلى داخل وأما الكسر الذي في /50b/ العرض فيجب أن يقوم العظمان على إستقامة[80] في غاية ما يمكن ويراعي ذلك من جهة وضع الأجزاء السليمة وينظر هل هي من هذا العظم محاذية لنظيرها من العظم الآخر ثم يجبر ويراعي الشظايا والزوائد والثلم.

السؤال السادس عشر—ما هي الأشياء التي تصلب الدشبد؟

الجواب—من القانون، هي النطولات القابضة اللطيفة والأضمدة التي تشبهها مثل طبيخ الآس ودهنه والطلاء بماء ورق الآس وحبه وطبيخ شجرة القرظ[81] وطبيخ أصل الدردار وطبيخ ورقه فإنه ملحم مصلب والضماد المتخذ[82] من الماش وخصوصاً إذا جعل فيه[83] زعفران ومر وعجن بشراب ريحاني جيد[84] جداً وقشور الطلع جيدة أيضاً.

السؤال السابع عشر—هل مدة الإنجبار في الأعضاء كلها مدة واحدة أو هي مختلفة بإختلاف الأعضاء فإن كانت مختلفة فما مثلها؟

الجواب—من القانون، مدة الإنجبار مختلفة من ذلك أن الأنف ينجبر[85] في عشرة أيام[86] والضلع في عشرين والذراع[87] وما يقرب منه في ثلاثين إلى أربعين والفخذ في خمسين وربما إمتدت المدة في الفخذ إلى <u>ثلاثة أشهر</u>[88] أو أربعة والساعد ربما إنجبر في ثمانية وعشرين يوماً وقد ذكر /51a/ ذلك في باب كسر الساعد.

السؤال الثامن عشر—ما هي الأسباب التي لأجلها يعسر جبر العظم؟

الجواب—كثرة التنظير أو كثرة حل الرباطات وربطها أو الإستعجال للحركة أو قلة الدم اللزج[89] في البدن أو قلة الدم مطلقاً ولذلك يقل إنجبار العظام في المبرودين والناقهين.

السؤال التاسع عشر—ما تقول في كسر العقب؟

الجواب—من القانون، إنكسار العقب صعب وعلاجه عسر وأكثر ما ينكسر إذا سقط الإنسان من موضع عال وربما عرض[90] رض عظيم مع سيلان دم إلى بطون العضل يجمد فيها ويؤدي[91] إلى أعراض عظيمة فإذا إنجبر العقب كان المشي عليه موجعاً وإذا لم ينجبر العقب على ما ينبغي بطل الإنتفاع به.

السؤال العشرون—كيف وضع العقب وما المنفعة به؟

الجواب—من القانون، هو موضوع تحت الكعب صلب مستدير إلى خلف ليقاوم المصاكات[92] والآفات مملس الأسفل ليحسن إستواء الوطء وإنطباق القدم على المستقر عند القيام وخلق مقداره إلى العظم ليستقل بحمل البدن وخلق مثلثاً إلى الإستطالة يدق يسيراً يسيراً /51b/ حتى ينتهي ويضمحل عند الأخمص إلى الوحشي ليكون تقعير الأخمص متدرجاً من خلف إلى متوسط[93].

الباب العاشر في مسائل من أصول هذه الصناعة

وهو عشرون مسألة

السؤال الأول—ما حجة من قال إن الإسطقسات[1] ليست أكثر من واحد؟

الجواب—من الشفاء لإبن سينا، إنه لما رأينا الأشياء الطبيعية يتغير بعضها إلى بعض وكل متغير فإن له شيئاً[2] ثابتاً في التغير هو الذي يتغير من حال إلى حال فيجب من ذلك أن يكون لجميع الأجسام الطبيعية شئ مشترك محفوظ هو عنصرها.

السؤال الثاني—ما حجة الذين قالوا إن الإسطقس هو النار؟

الجواب—من الشفاء، وذلك أنهم يرون أن النار كبيرة الجوهر ثم إستحقروا حجم الأرض والماء والهواء في جنبته[3] إذ السموات المشعة[4] والكواكب المضيئة كلها عندهم نارية وحكموا بأن الجرم الأكبر مقداراً هو الأولى أن يكون عنصراً وخصوصاً ولا جسم[5] أصرف في طبيعته من النار وأن الحرارة هي المبثوثة[6] في الكائنات كلها وما الهواء إلا[7] نار مفترة[8] ببرد البخار وما البخار إلا ماء هو /52a/ متحلل وما الماء إلا نار متكثفة[9] وهواء كثيفاً[10] ولو كان للبرد عنصر يتصور به ولم يكن البرد أمراً عرضياً كان في العناصر بارد برده في وزان[11] شدة الحر[12] النار.

السؤال الثالث—ما[13] حجة الذين قالوا إن الإسطقس واحد وهو الماء؟

الجواب—من الشفاء، إنهم قالوا إن معنّى الرطوبة أثبت في الهوائية[14] في الماء فلذلك[15] مطاوعته للمعنى المذكور أشد وما الماء إلا هواء متكاثف[16] والمتكاثف أقرب[17] إلى اليبس منه إلى التخلخل[18] وأما الأرض فهي ما عرض له التكاثف الشديد كما نراه من إنعقاد[19] المياه السائلة حجارة وأما النار فليست هي إلا هواء إشتدت[20] به الحرارة فرام سمواً.

السؤال الرابع—ما حجة من قال إن إسطقسات الأجسام هي إثنان وهما النار والأرض؟

الجواب—من الشفاء لإبن سينا، قالوا إن سائر الإسطقسات تستحيل آخر الأمر إلى هذين الطرفين والطرفان لا يستحيلان إلى إسطقسات أخرى خارجة عنهما فهما الإسطقسان ولذلك هما بالغان[21] في[22] الخفة والثقل والآخران يقصران عنهما إذ[23] لا حركة إسطقسة[24] إلا إثنان[25] فالأغلب في الإثنين[26] هو الإسطقس والنار والأرض بالقياس إلى غيرهما[27] أغلب منهما ثم الهواء /52b/ نار جامدة[28] مفترة مثقلة[29] بالماء المتبخر والماء أرض متحللة[30] سائلة[31] خالطتها نارية فهي أخف من الأرض.

السؤال الخامس—ما حجة من قال إن الإسطقسات إثنان وهما الأرض والماء؟

الجواب—يرون أن حاجة المركبات إلى الرطب واليابس وكما أنها تحتاج إلى الرطب ليقبل التخليق لذلك تحتاج إلى اليابس ليحفظ التخليق فإن الرطب

سهل القبول سهل الخلع واليابس صعب القبول صعب الخلع فإذا تخمر اليابس بالرطب إستفاد المركب من الرطب حسن مطاوعة[32] للتخليق ومن اليابس شدة إستحفاظ[33] له فاليابس والرطب في المشاهدة هما الأرض والماء لا غير.

السؤال السادس—ما هو الشئ الذي إذا إعتبر ظهر أن الإسطقسات الأربعة يتكون بعضها من بعض؟

الجواب—من الشفاء لإبن سينا حيث يقول: وإذا إعتبر المعتبر صادف[34] النبات[35] والحيوان المتكون في حيز الأرض مستمدة من الأرض ومن الماء ومن الهواء ووجدها[36] يتم بإتحاد[37] المنضج والأرض تفيد الكائن تماسكاً[38] وحفظاً للتشكيل والتخطيط[39] والماء يفيد الكائن سهولة قبول للتخليق والتشكيل[40] يستمسك جوهر الماء بعد سيلانه بمخالطة الأرض ويستمسك جوهر الأرض عن تشتته بمخالطة الماء والهواء والنار /53a/ يكسران صرفة[41] هذين ويفيدانهما[42] إعتدال الإمتزاج والهواء يخلخل ويفيد وجود المنافذ والمسام والنار تنضج وتطبخ وتجمع فقد ظهر أنها يتكون بعضها من بعض.

السؤال السابع—ما هو المزاج؟

الجواب—من القانون حيث يقول: المزاج كيفية تحدث[43] من تفاعل كيفيات متضادة[44] موجودة في عناصر متصغرة الأجزاء لتماس[45] أكثر كل واحد منها أكثر الآخرإذا تفاعلت بقواها بعضها في بعض حدث من[46] جملتها كيفية متشابهة[47] في جميعها هي المزاج.

السؤال الثامن—ما هو النضج وهل له أصناف أم لا؟

الجواب—من الشفاء، النضج هو إحالة من الحرارة للجسم ذي الرطوبة إلى موافقة الغاية المقصودة وهذا على أصناف منه نضج نوع الشئ ومنه نضج الغذاء ومنه نضج الفضل[48] وقد يقال لما كان بالصناعة أيضاً نضج فأما نضج نوع الشئ فمثل نضج الثمرة والفاعل لهذا النضج موجود في جوهر النضيج ويحيل رطوبته إلى قوام موافق للغاية المقصودة في كونه وإنما يتم فيما يولد المثل أن يصير بحيث يولد المثل وأما نضج الغذاء فليس هو على سبيل النضج الذي لنوع الشئ وذلك لأن نضج الغذاء يفسد جوهر الغذاء ويحيله إلى مشاكلة طبيعة جوهر[49] /53b/ المغتذى وفاعل هذا النضج[50] ليس موجوداً في جوهر ما ينضج بل في جوهر ما يستحيل إليه لكنه مع ذلك إحالة من الحرارة للرطوبة إلى موافقة الغاية المقصودة التي هي إفادة بدل ما يتحلل والإسم الخاص بهذا النضج هو الهضم وأما نضج الفضل من حيث هو فضل أعنى من حيث لا ينتفع به في أن يغذوا فهو مفارق للنوعين الأولين فإن هذا النضج إحالة الرطوبة إلى قوام ومزاج يسهل به دفعها إما بتغليظ قوامه إن كان المانع عن دفعه شدة سيلانه ورقته وإما بترقيقه إن كان المانع شدة غلظه وإما بتقطيعه إن كان المانع لزوجته.

السؤال التاسع—ما العلة[51] في أن فسطاط مصر قليل المطر كثير الندي[52]؟

الجواب—من كتاب النجاة في المسائل، قالوا إن البخار إذا صار إلى مواضع عادمة[53] لما يحبس النجار ويحصره ويكثفه فيتعدا أيضاً[54] البخار فإذا جاوزها إلى موضع آخر حتى يلقى ما يحصره ويحبسه ومتى كان موضعاً متكشفاً من الجبال وأرضه تبخر بخاراً كثيراً لقبولها لذلك من حر الشمس فإذا غربت

الشمس عنه برد فتحلل بالليل ندى كثيراً وقد يكون موضع عادم للبخار لأنه لا يقبل ذلك ومواضع كثيرة البخار ولها جبال تحصر بخارها حتى يتكاثف فتكون كثيرة المطر وفسطاط مصر من جهة شمالها عادم للجبال الشوامخ وأكثر ما يسيل إليها البخار[55] من الجنوب /54a/ إلى الشمال من جهة بحر الحبشة وأيضاً فإن نيل مصر يفيض على جميع أرضها ويقيم عليها زماناً فإذا نقص إرتد[56] ذلك الفاضل من الزائد إلى بطن الأرض فتقبله تلك[57] الأرض لكثرة إقامته على وجهها فيكثر ما يرتفع من أرضها في كل يوم من البخار بحر الشمس فإذا غربت عنها الشمس صار ذلك البخار غيماً فيتحلل بالليل لتخلخله وضعفه وقلة كثافته، قال: فهذه العلة يقل مطرها ويكثر نداها.

السؤال العاشر—كم هي الأشياء التي تتم وتكمل بها[58] صناعة الطب؟

الجواب—من المدخل إلى علم الطب لقسطا إبن لوقا حيث يقول: إنها عشرة، الأول البحث عن الأصول التي كان عنها بدن الإنسان، الثاني البحث عن الأمزاج والتراكيب الذي تركبت عليه تلك الأصول التي كان عنها بدن الإنسان، الثالث البحث عن عدد الأعضاء وخلقتها وتركيبها، الرابع البحث عن قواها وأفعالها، الخامس البحث عن منافعها التي خلقت لها، السادس البحث عن حفظ صحتها، السابع البحث[59] عما يحدث في واحد منها من الأمراض والأعراض، الثامن البحث عن علل الأمراض الحادثة بها، التاسع البحث عن العلامات الدالة عليها، العاشر البحث عن التدابير المشفية لها الدافعة عنها /54b/ الأمراض الحادثة بها.

السؤال الحادي عشر—كم هي أصناف الأعضاء المتشابهة الأجزاء؟

الجواب—من الملكي، سبعة أصناف الأول صنف العظام والغضاريف، الثاني صنف العصب والوتر، الثالث صنف العروق غير الضوارب، الرابع صنف العروق الضوارب، الخامس صنف اللحم المفرد والغدد والشحم، السادس صنف الجلد والأغشية، السابع صنف الأظفار والشعر.

السؤال الثاني عشر—كم هي الأفعال الضرورية في قوام الحيوان؟

الجواب—من طبيعيات الشفاء، ثلاثة، فعل تغذية البدن ويصدر عن القوّة الطبيعية وفعل تغذية الروح وتعديلها ويصدر عن القوّة الحيوانية وفعل الحس والحركة ويصدر عن القوّة النفسانية.

السؤال الثالث عشر—ما هو السبب البادئ والسابق والواصل؟

الجواب—من شرح أغلوقن لعلي إبن رضوان، أما البادئ فهو ما أثر في البدن أثراً وبطل والسابق هو ما جمع في البدن مادة أو فعل سوء مزاج مثل كثرة الأخلاط عن التملئ باالشرب والواصل يسمى الماسك مثل عفونة الأخلاط فإنها سبب ماسك للحمى يدوم بدوامها /55a/.

السؤال الرابع عشر—ما هو الفصل الرابع والخمسون من المقالة الرابعة من فصول إبقراط[60] وما معناه؟

الجواب—أما الفصل فقول إبقراط: من عرض له حمى محرقة وسعال كثير يابس ثم كان تهيجه له يسير فإنه لا يكاد يعطش فسرّه جالينوس السعال اليابس قد يكون من خراج رديء يحدث في آلات التنفس وقد يكون من خشونة في الحلق

وقد يكون من رطوبة رقيقة يسيرة تجري فيه وأى هذه الأسباب كان فإن قصبة الرئة كأنها تبتل[61] به ولذلك يقل العطش.

السؤال الخامس عشر—ما هو الفصل الخامس والستون من المقالة الخامسة من فصول إبقراط وما معناه؟

الجواب—أما الفصل فهو إذا حدثت خراجات عظيمة خبيثة ثم لم يكن يظهر معها ورم فالبلية عظيمة فسّره جالينوس يعني بالخراجات الخبيثة[62] الكائنة في رؤوس العضل أو في نهائها[63] وخاصة ما كان من العضل الغالب عليه العصب لأن رؤوس العضل[64] يتصل بالعصب ومن أطرافها تنبت الأوتار وقوله بلية عظيمة لأنه لا يؤمن أن يكون الأخلاط التي تنصب إلى الخراجات بسبب الوجع الحادث في القرحة تجري إليه لا محالة فيعظم الضرب.

السؤال السادس عشر—كم هي القوانين /55b/ التي يتعرف منها علل الأعضاء[65] الباطنة؟

الجواب—من المقالة الأولى من جوامع التعرف لجالينوس حيث يقول: ستة، أولها ما ينال الأفعال من المضار، الثاني الأشياء التي تبرز[66] وتخرج، الثالث الأورام الحادثة، الرابع الوجع، الخامس الأعراض الخاصة، السادس المشتركة في العلة.

السؤال السابع عشر—كم هي أصناف ما يعرض في البدن من الأشياء الخارجة عن الطبيعة؟

الجواب—من المقالة الثانية من حيلة البرء لجالينوس، أربعة، أحدها نفس

الفعل الذي نزلت به الآفة والضرر، الثاني في البنية والهيئة الفاعلة، الثالث السبب الفاعل لهذه البنية والهيئة، الرابع العرض اللازم التابع لهذه الهيئة والبنية فليسم[67] بنية البدن وهيئة المضرورة والعائقة للفعل مرضاً ويسمى ما يتبع ذلك عرضاً ويسمى الشئ الفاعل المتمم لهذه البنية والهيئة سبباً.

السؤال الثامن عشر—كيف يسخن الماء البارد وكيف يبرد الماء الحار؟

الجواب—من المقالة الأولى من الأدوية المفردة لجالينوس حيث يقول: الماء البارد كثيراً ما يكون سبباً /56a/ لتراجع الحرارة من طريق تبريد الخلط[68] وجمعه إياه والماء الحار كثيراً ما يبرد من طريق تحليلة الخلط الذي يسخن.

السؤال التاسع عشر—كم هي الشروط[69] التي إذا إجتمعت أثر السبب البادئ في البدن مرضاً؟

الجواب—من الأصول لإبن رضوان، ثلاثة، أحدها أن يكون البدن متهيأً لحدوث ذلك المرض أعنى قابلاً لتأثير ذلك السبب، الثاني أن يكون مقدار السبب مقداراً كثيراً أو قوّته شديدة لتمكنه بذلك أن يغير البدن، الثالث أن يبقى ملاق[70] للبدن زماناً في مثله يمكن أن يتغير عنه البدن.

السؤال العشرون—كم هي الأسباب في قبول العضو القابل؟

الجواب—سبعة، الأول إجتماع فضله في العضو الدافع، الثاني قوّة الدافع، الثالث ضعف القابل، الرابع سعة المجاري، الخامس تخلخل جرم القابل أسفل فيرجحن[71] المادة إلى أسفل، السابع[72] ضيق المجاري التي يدفع القابل فضوله

فيها.

فنسأل[73] اللّه العظيم أن يلهمنا لطاعته ويسلكنا طريق رضاه في عبادته ويجمعنا في دار كرامته وأن يرزقنا شفاعة محمد سيد الرسل صلى اللّه عليه وعلى آله[74] وأصحابه الطاهرين[75] أجمعين،[76] إن شاء اللّه عز وجل[77].

الملاحظات

Abbreviations: B = Bursa manuscript, C = Cairo manuscript, V = Vienna manuscript, PE = published edition of the work cited in the answer.

المقدمة

1) In B followed by رب يسر يا كريم, in C by وبه الإغاثة . 2) Lacking in C. 3) Lacking in C. 4) In V عليت. 5) In V عموق. 6) Lacking in C. 7) In C followed by الصاحب. 8) In B يخيو. 9) In B and C تقلع, in V يقلع. 10) In C and V استعلا. 11) In V نشج. 12) In V followed by والتايل. 13) In V قول. 14) In C followed by لا زالت. 15) In V يلوح. 16) In V اشغلنا. 17) In B and C لا تناه. 18) In B and C مخلدا. 19) In B سليل, in C سيل, and in V سل. 20) In V نظاره. 21) In V ناجية . 22) In V marginal note الجبلي تذكرة هو الكبش . 23) In C الأفعي. 24) Underlined words lacking in V. 25) In B, C, and V فياخذه. 26) In V ابن سيني. 27) In B ملازم للقراءه, in V ملازم القراة. 28) In C المرضى الذين يعالجهم. 29) In C العلل التى يتولى علاجها. 30) Lacking in V. 31) Lacking in B and V. 32) In B and C الفقه. 33) In C رضي اللّه عنه. 34) Lacking in C. 35) In C عن. 36) In B and C يتطاول. 37) Underlined words lacking in C. 38) Lacking in B and V.

الملاحظات

الباب الأول

1) Underlined words lacking in V. 2) In B and C قال. 3) In PE نبضه نبضاً. 4) In PE followed by البتة. 5) In PE الهموم. 6) In PE ويمكن من ذلك ان. 7) Lacking in PE. 8) In PE المعشوق throughout. 9) In PE والحيلة في. 10) Lacking in PE. 11) In PE يذكر. 12) In PE يكون. 13) In PE نبضه. 14) In PE بذلك. 15) In C فصنف. 16) Rephrased in PE. 17) In PE شبه المنقطع. 18) Lacking in PE. 19) In PE علمت انه. 20) In V خمسة precedes الجواب. 21) Sic. 22) Lacking in C. 23) In V المروحات. 24) In B and C في ان in place of the previous two words. 25) In PE followed by بينهما. 26) In PE حال. 27) In PE followed by وفي المقدار. 28) In PE كالتليفية. 29) In PE followed by وقد تكون غير. 30) As previous note. 31) In C نسبة, in PE نسب. 32) In V ابن. 33) In PE words reversed. 34) Lacking in B and C. 35) In C فان النبض, in PE و instead of ف. 36) In B and C ثم. 37) In PE followed by ايضاً. 38) In PE فان. 39) Lacking in PE. 40) In PE followed by الإجتماع. 41) In PE يكون. 42) In PE followed by الى الخارج والى مبدئه لذلك. 43) In PE followed by بالنائم. 44) In PE followed by التى لا تحسن هذا. 45) In PE النائم. 46) In PE followed by ميلاً. 47) In PE followed by ورجع الى حاله الطبيعى. 48) In PE فاما. 49) In PE followed by دفعة. 50) In PE ثم يعود له نبض عظيم سريع متواتر مختلف. 51) In PE

يسرع الى الإعتدال. 52) In V مائل. 53) In C بسبب. 54) In C اذا. 55) Lacking in B and C. 56) In V سريع. 57) Underlined words lacking in C. 58) In C ثم كان in place of ان لم يكن. 59) In C من. 60) In PE يكون. 61) Lacking in PE here and in the two instances that follow. 62) In PE كيفيته. 63) In B and C الجز العملي. 64) Lacking in C. 65) In PE الضعيفة. 66) Lacking in PE. 67) Underlined words lacking in B and C. 68) In B وكيف ذلك, lacking in C. 69) In C followed by حيث يقول. 70) In PE الحوامل. 71) In PE نبض صاحبه. 72) In PE differently phrased. 33) In B, V, and PE موجى عريض لين. 74) In V الطبيعي which is preceded by اللحمي. 75) Partial summary of PE. 76) In PE followed by اذا. 77) In PE وان. 78) In PE هاج.

الباب الثاني

1) Lacking in B and C. 2) Lacking in B and C. 3) In C and V بخاصة. 4) Lacking in C. 5) Lacking in B and C. 6) In C كان. 7) Lacking in B and C. 8) In PE المتعلق. 9) In PE الراسب. 10) In C الدم. 11) In B, C, and V راحة. 12) In B الجريات and in V الجزويات. 13) In B, C, and V followed by والتى. 14) In C على. 15) In B, C, and V followed by إما. 16) In V هظم. 17) In PE سدداً بل ان. 18) Lacking in C, and in V ابن. 19) In PE فلذلك. 20) Underlined words lacking in V. 21) Lacking in PE. 22) and 23) In PE

او. 24) In V دسيسى. 25) Lacking in PE. 26) In PE و منه and for all the following و that are not lacking. 27) In B and C دمي. 28) and 29) Lacking in PE. 19) Underlined words lacking in B, C and PE.

الباب الثالث

1) In C غبية. 2) In B راجية, this and the previous word are separate items in B, C, and V but are together in PE. 3) Lacking in C. 4) In B, C, V, and PE عشيية. 5) In V لحمية. 6) In V السب, in PE المياء القابضة. 7) In B and V غدائية. 8) In V نافص. 9) In B and C نوابها, in V بواتها. 10) In C ابطاوه. 11) In V نقصايا. 12) In V يحور. 13) In V يقرها. 14) Underlined words lacking in C. 15) In B and C ينذر, in V يتدر. 16) In V يقضى. 17) In C الثالث. 18) In B المشبعه and in C المسيعه. 19) In C اللحم. 20) Lacking in C. 21) In C الهوى. 22) In C المتاد. 23) In B and C المرض. 24) In C السواد. 25) In V رقيق مايى. 26) In B and C اثنى. 27) In B and C ما. 28) Lacking in B and V. 29) Lacking in B and V. 30) In V تحمر. 31) In V الشا. 32) In V يزيد. 33) In C البتة. 34) In B and C تزيد, in V يزيد. 35) In B and C تزيده. 36) In B and C الحالة. 37) In V بزيد. 38) In V بضاعط. 39) In V بادا وظاهر. 40) In V ا. 41) Lacking in B and C. 42) In V بودي. 43) In B and V انا. 44) In B معمورة. 45) In B and C تدرك. 46) Lacking in B and V. 47) In V يترك. 48) In V الاجراء. 49) In B and C فاعلتين. 50)

Lacking in C. 51) In B and C المنفعلتين. 52) In V الاجراء. 53) In V فاحدث. 54) In V الثانية. 55) Lacking in B and V. 56) In C البرد. 57) In V يكون. 58) Lacking in C. 59) In B and C الفاعلتين. 60) Lacking in C. 61) In B and C المتفعلتين. 62) In V النقص. 63) In B المرض. 64) In B and C دفعة. 65) Underlined words lacking in V. 66) In C يعنى. 67) In V حوده. 68) In C المرض. 69) Lacking in C. 70) Lacking in V. 71) In V اندر. 72) In V حشا. 73) In B and C له. 74) In V البواب. 75) In V سوب. 76) In V بابى. 77) In V سطى. 78) In C this word preceded by باكى. 79) In V بسغى. 80) In C بتنق. 81) In V البغر. 82) In V اندار. 83) In C جرح. 84) In V اليوم. 85) In B and C الاول. 86) In B and C الاقوى. 87) Lacking in V. 88) In C الحر لرابع. 89) In B تكون. 90) In B and C العشرين. 91) In V الثلثون. 92) In V followed by و. 93) In B and V من. 94) In V عشرين. 95) In V ثلثون. 96) In V انقصا. 97) In V بالجراحات. 98) In V بسحف. 99) In B and C الست. 100) In V العشرون. 101) In C followed by بحرانه. 102) B and C lack question number twenty.

الباب الرابع

1) Underlined words on margin in B, lacking in V. 2) In B and C انقضت, in V انقصت. 3) In V بجراحات. 4) In PE ستحدث. 5) In PE followed by مادة. 6) Lacking in PE. 7) In PE تنضج. 8) Lacking in PE. 9) In PE العينين.

10) In PE مرض. 11) Lacking in PE. 12) In B and C تدل. 13) In PE العليل. 14) In B and C الماوف, in V الماووف, in PE المؤف. 15) In PE إذا كانت. 16) In PE فيحترق. 17) In PE سريع. 18) Lacking in PE. 19) In PE بالقوّة. 20) In B and V سب. 21) In V بكلسها. 22) In PE دفع. 23) In PE فعند ذلك تسقط. 24) In C القوى. 25) In PE على ذلك. 26) In V المانه. 27) Underlined words lacking in C, summary of PE. 28) In C ثوارن. 29) In PE غلطه. 30) In PE ووجود. 31) In PE حصر. 32) In PE اسفل البطن. 33) In PE وفقد ل. 34) In PE بل. 35) In PE ظهر. 36) and 37) Lacking in PE. 38) In B and V عسه. 39) In PE ابيض. 40) In C احمرا رقيقا ابيضا. 41) In B and C العرق. 42) In PE صار. 43) In B الرحمه, in C الرحعه, in V الوحيه, in PE الموجبة. 44) In PE كان. 45) In PE يجب. 46) In PE قارن. 47) In PE الشفة. 48) In PE اذ. 49) In V باقص. 50) In PE حكم انه. 51) In PE خصوصاً. 52) In C ان كان. 53) In C followed by يكون. 54) and 55) In PE او. 56) In PE followed by انبساطاً. 57) In V احل, in PE وحك. 58) In PE خصوصاً. 59) In PE على ان. 60) In C indefinite. 61) In V سحرن. 62) In PE بالرعاف. 63) In PE بالتسخين. 64) Lacking in PE. 65) In PE إذ. 66) In B and C لتسكين. 67) In PE دليل. 68) In PE الذرب (diarrhea). 69) In PE يكون. 70) Lacking in C. 71) In V برعح. 72) In PE على السلامة. 73) In V صمم. 74) In B and V بعقب. 75) In PE المرارى. 76) In V لذلك. 77) In PE متى. 78) In PE السبب. 79) In PE ذلك ضد ما قلته. 80)

Lacking in PE. 81) In PE الأسفل. 82) In PE مادة.

الباب الخامس

1) Underlined words lacking in V. 2) Lacking in C. 3) In C and V المرادة. 4) Underlined words lacking in C. 5) In V يحل. 6) This and the previous word are reversed in B. 7) In B النار بكعن, in C النار بكين, and in V والنار بكعين. 8) In B الشرخشت, in C السيرخشت. 9) In B and C اللادن. 10) In V النوار. 11) In B and C السرو (cypress tree), in V الشرق. 12) Unidentified. In B النار بلون, in C الناربكون, and in V النار يكمن. 13) In B الشرخشت, in C السيرخشت. 14) In V بهرا. 15) In C يخرجه. 16) Underlined words lacking in C. 17) In V نقيا. 18) In C العلك. 19) Lacking in C. 20) On margin in B, lacking in V. 21) Lacking in B and V. 22) In V الل. 23) In C يتركم. 24) In V يسط. 25) In V فتعلب. 26) In V محتص. 27) In C الدليل. 28) In C القنديل. 29) In V الصيد. 30) Underlined words lacking in C. 31) In B فيسقط. 32) In V الهوى. 33) Lacking in B and V. 34) Lacking in PE. 35) In C فسقيب, in V فراب. 36) In B and C علة, in PE إن. 37) In PE لان. 38) In B and C السوداوى. 39) In PE followed by أو. 40) In C الدا. 41) In B and C هذا. 42) In V بهسة. 43) In V ترك. 44) In C فوق. 45) In C يخرج. 46) In C يلبس. 47) In V يزيد.

48) Lacking in C. 49) Lacking in C. 50) In PE followed by البحر. 51) In PE أُسطوكودوس. 52) In PE إدخر. 53) In B and C ايل, in PE أثل (tamarisk). 54) In V بانويح. 55) In PE باذرنجبة. 56) In PE كادي (screw pine). 57) Lacking in PE. 58) In PE جوز (walnut). 59) In PE followed by قنبيط (cauliflower). 60) In V كرمروغب, in PE و is lacking. 61) In B كسوب, in V كسوف, in PE كشوت. 62) In B and C كل سى, lacking in PE. 63) In V منعه. 64) In PE نيلج. 65) In PE followed by الخشب (wood). 66) In V يحكب, lacking in PE. 67) This and the previous word are reversed in C. 68) In PE سرجس. 69) In PE فسطق. 70) In PE as two items فاونية فو, the second word being grand valerian. 71) In PE قلب (lithospermum officinale). 72) In PE ربوب (?). 73) In C شيبه, in PE followed by شاهتريج (fumitory). 74) In PE شاهشبروم. 75) Lacking in PE. 76) In V جندروس. 77) Lacking in PE. 78) In PE جوز جندم as one item (?). 79) In B and V لسان، موز in place of لسان ثور. 80) In PE ملوك preceded by موز (plantain ?). 81) Lacking in C. 82) In PE followed by بليلج (terminalia bellerica). 83) In B and C اسطر اطيقوس, in V اسطر اطفوس, in PE اسطير اطيفوس. 84) In B and V بردا, in PE برذي. 85) Lacking in C, in PE دخان. 86) In B, C, and PE ديساقوس. 87) In V حرار الصحر. 88) In PE مقل مكي as one item. 89) In PE نجم (cynodon dactylon) followed by

سندروس (sandarach). 90) In PE سذر وهو النبق. 91) In B and C سادوران. 92) In PE عليس. 93) In B غزا, in V عرا. 94) In PE اسفاناك. 95) Lacking in PE. 96) In PE نيلوفر. 97) In PE قراسيا. 98) In B, C, and PE خبازي. 99) In PE followed by الطيب as one item. 100) In PE ابونوس. 101) In B and V اربل, in C انزيل, in PE ابرنج (?). 102) In PE اناغاليس. 103) In V الاسقافس, in PE الاسفاقش. 104) In PE برنجمشك وهو الحبق (mint). 105) In V جلون, in PE followed by جوز القي (nux vomica?). 106) In PE الكور. 107) In PE حمحم. 108) In B and C قفر. 109) Lacking in PE. 110) In V كماقيطوس. 111) In PE مصطكى. 112) In PE سعدى. 113) In V given as two items سقولو، فندريون. 114) In PE فاجرة. 115) In C زراوند (Aristolochia). 116) In PE بهمنان. 117) In PE العصافير. 118) In V معاذ, in PE معاد. 119) In PE بارس. 120) Lacking in PE. 121) In PE followed by عربي. 122) In C and PE خيار (purging cassia tree). 123) Lacking in B and C. 124) In C ثلاثون. 125) In PE انجذان. 126) In PE افيثمون. 127) In PE بسبايج. 128) In C سك and PE lacks the و before this and the previous word. 129) Lacking in PE. 130) In PE دخون. 131) In C and PE دوقو. 132) Lacking in PE. 133) In PE خرشف. 134) In B and C خماMالاون. 135) In B, C, and V لوفس, and in V a separate item from the previous one, lacking in PE. 136) In PE مالش. 137) Lacking in PE. 138) In B and V حب بان. 139) Lacking in C. 140) In

V نيل. 141) In V اوطى, in PE حما اقطى. 142) In B and C يربطون. 143) In C كراوية, in V كزاويا, in PE كروية. 144) In PE كبر مر (?). 145) In C مومية. 146) In B and V ينبوته, in PE بنتشه (?). 147) In PE followed by صفر. 148) In B and C اسعلسوس, lacking in PE. 149) In PE فنجكست. 150) In PE فودنج. 151) In B and V قلقلمونه, in PE فلفلموية. 152) This and the previous word are separate items in V. 153) Lacking in V. 154) In PE صغير. 155) Lacking in V. 156) In B and V قسطرن, in PE قسطرن (?). 157) In PE خلنجان. 158) Lacking in PE. 159) In PE الاس (myrtle). 160) In PE عصا.

الباب السادس

1) In B and C الغرض throughout. 2) This and the previous word are reversed in C. 3) In B, C, and V followed by به. 4) Lacking in C. 5) In C لذلك. 6) Lacking in V. 7) Underlined words lacking in C. 8) In C الشئين. 9) In C الهوى. 10) In B and C كتب. 11) In V بمرله. 12) In B and C زذنا, in V زدنا. 13) In V يداوى. 14) In B and C اما. 15) In V تراعا. 16) In PE يجذب. 17) In PE يحبس. 18) In V عن. 19) In V الندين. 20) In PE التبعيد. 21) In V الحلال. 22) In PE أو. 23) In B and C مضر. 24) In PE بأخرى فنضطر أن نركب معه. 25) In PE خلطنا. 26) In PE مضرة. 27) Lacking in PE. 28) In PE به. 29) In PE كإختلاط. 30) Lacking in C. 31) In C الامزجة.

32) In PE أو. 33) In PE يستعمل. 34) In PE أن يركب. 35) Lacking in PE. 36) In PE احتيج. 37) In PE لم يكن. 38) Lacking in PE. 39) In PE يستعمل. 40) In PE يرقق أو يدقق. 41) In PE تستعمل. 42) Lacking in PE. 43) In V يحل. 44) In V يذاب. 45) In V مستحكم. 46) In V اللون. 47) In V مداواه. 48) In PE بمنع. 49) This and the previous word are reversed in C. 50) In PE الملائمة. 51) In B and C العضل. 52) In B, C, and V الهواء، والبلد. 53) In PE وتعقبه. 54) In PE ربما. 55) In PE يجب. 56) In PE followed by من المستفرغ. 57) In PE يندفع. 58) In PE يجزم. 59) In B, C, and V الإستفراغ. 60) In PE followed by فيها. 61) Lacking in C. 62) In PE البدار. 63) In B, C, and PE اولى. 64) In PE متداخلة. 65) In PE يحرك. 66) In V احد. 67) In PE بالتى لا تبرئ الثانية. 68) In C بدون. 69) In PE برئه. 70) In PE followed by سوء. 71) In PE الثانية. 72) In PE وعلاج سببها. 73) In PE الثالثة. 74) In PE اذا. 75) In PE حمى مطبقة سوناخس. 76) In PE سوناخس. 77) Underlined words lacking in V. 78) In PE يغلبه. 79) In PE followed by فصد. 80) In B, C, and V للمرض. 81) Lacking in B and V. 82) Lacking in C. 83) Lacking in V. 84) Lacking in C. 85) Lacking in V. 86) This and the previous two words lacking in C. 87) Lacking in C. 88) Lacking in V. 89) In V عن. 90) Lacking in V. 91) Lacking in V. 92) Lacking in V. 93) This word repeated twice in V. 94) In C المختلطة. 95) In C المزاج. 96) In B الايارج فيقرا, in C ايادج فيقرا, in V الارياح القمر. 97) In C فريطس. 98) In

V المحرق. 99) In C السود, in V السودائي. 100) In V الاختلاع. 101) Number sixty-five is lacking in B and C. 102) Number sixty-seven is lacking in C. 103) Given as number sixty-eight in C. 104) In B بخمل. 105) In V بحدده. 106) In V بحدب. 107) In V الحرارة. 108) In V البحاد. 109) In V البحامة. 110) In PE وتحتاج ان. 111) Summary of PE. 112) In PE للخلط قطعت. 113) In B and V الغدا. 114) In PE قاصرة. 115) In PE followed by المزاج. 116) In PE followed by لها. 117) In PE نعشت. 118) In B and V الغدا. 119) In B and V قصد. 120) In PE تعجل. 121) In PE تقتصر. 122) In PE لا باس بها. 123) In B باخرة. 124) In PE بعد ذلك فاستفرغ. 125) In V يعد. 126) In PE على مثل ماء الشعير وماء العسل اطعامه فانه يجب ان تقتصب بالمفلوج فى اول ما يظهر. 127) Lacking in B, C, and V. 128) In V followed by كلما. 129) In B, C, and V من. 130) In all تضحل. 131) In PE اصلح. 132) Words reversed in PE. 133) In PE القوانين المذكورة بالمشروبات. 134) In C and PE حقن. 135) In PE حادة. 136) Summary of PE. 137) In V بدنا. 138) In PE و. 139) In V حنس. 140) In PE تحبس. 141) Lacking in PE. 142) In PE وان. 143) In PE كراهيته. 144) Lacking in PE. 145) Items reversed in PE. 146) In PE الخلاء. 147) In PE ياكل. 148) In PE فيزول. 149) In PE المبردات المرطبة. 150) In PE followed by فيه. 151) In PE تنقية. 152) In PE يعالج. 153) In V ضادها.

154) In B and C يتحلل. 155) In B and V سحف. 156) In V كثافه. 157) In C followed by كالعقارب (like scorpions). 158) In V العشه. 159) In PE يزاد. 160) In PE followed by له. 161) In PE نحو الفوق. 162) In PE ايذاء. 163) In PE يرخى. 164) In PE يوافقها. 165) In PE الغير. 166) In B and V لذلك. 167) In V نسسنع. 168) In PE للمعدة. 169) In B and C مضر, in PE فيضر. 170) In PE عظيماً. 171) In C بالاضعاف. 172) Lacking in V. 173) In V سنى. 174) and 175) In PE الطعام. 176) In PE الشرب ل. 177) and 178) In PE و. 179) Lacking in PE. 180) In PE followed by للكبد. 181) In B and V الامتيار. 182) In PE followed by و. 183) Lacking in C. 184) In PE تمزجه بشراب ولا تبرده. 185) In PE تغب غباً. 186) In PE تمصه. 187) Lacking in PE. 188) In PE اللزوجات.

الباب السابع

1) In C سوالا. 2) In C عن. 3) In B and C من. 4) Lacking in C. 5) In B and V التي. 6) In V جزؤ. 7) This and the previous word are feminine in PE. 8) Lacking in PE. 9) As in note six. 10) In PE الباصرة. 11) In PE الجليديتين. 12) In PE في. 13) In PE الباصرة. 14) As in note six. 15) In B and V من كره. 16) In PE الجليديتين. 17) Lacking in B and C. 18) In PE الباطنة التى. 19) In PE إليها. 20) In B and V ومملها, in C فتنقلها, in PE

فنقلتها. 21) In C فلا. 22) In PE ينمحى. 23) In PE فتجزأت. 24) In B and C كما. 25) Lacking in C. 26) Lacking in V. 27) In V العتمه. 28) In C سهل. 29) Lacking in B, C, and V. 30) In PE أو. 31) In PE رؤى. 32) This and the previous word are reversed in C. 33) In V نعما. 34) In PE قلع. 35) In PE فاما. 36) In PE followed by والحركات. 37) In PE مثل. 38) Lacking in PE. 39) Underlined words on margin in B, lacking in V. 40) Word on margin in B, lacking in V, in PE يضره. 41) through 45) Lacking in PE. 46) In C and PE المبخرة, in V فالمحره. 47) In PE شبت. 48) In C بحيث لا يفسد هضمها, PE like C but without لا. 49) In B اعص, in C اعض. 50) In PE الطبقة. 51) In PE كانت. 52) Lacking in B and C. 53) In PE منها بالنهار. 54) In B اليبس, in C الينس, in V السن. 55) In B and C من. 56) and 57) In PE يعجز. 58) In PE ما. 59) In B الاتصال. 60) In C and PE الصرف. 61) Lacking in B, C, and V. 62) In V المعدة. 63) In PE لها تجفيف غير كثير و. 64) In V فانها. 65) In B بعلاجة, in C بالعلاج. 66) In PE فابدأ. 67) In PE تعالج. 68) In V بزبله. 69) In PE يغن. 70) In PE الصائب. 71) In C لجحت, in PE underlined words خبيثة لحجة. 72) In PE النافذ. 73) In PE و. 74) Lacking in B and V. 75) In B and V preceded by ما. 76) In B and C انتقعت, in V انفقت. 77) In B تنضر (?), in C تنضرز, in V تنصر. 78) In V نشح. 79) In B and V اربعة. 80) In V لغط. 81) In C رطوبة. 82) In B and V حفوفها, in C حفافها. 83) Lacking in C. 84) In V التى هى. 85) In PE بخار يتصاعد. 86)

In PE فيرى. 87) In PE ربما. 88) In V بعض. 89) In V بعصر. 90) Lacking in PE. 91) In PE ل. 92) In PE التحلل. 93) Lacking in C. 94) Lacking in B and C. 95) In V لبغرى, in PE الثانية أنها تغرى بلزوجتها. 96) In V لرلحس. 97) In PE حجارية. 98) In PE القى. 99) In B, C, and V فإختارات. 100) In B and V بياض. 101) Lacking in PE. 102) In PE يعرض. 103) In PE البرودة واليبوسة. 104) In PE followed by يعرض. 105) In PE يعرض. 106) Lacking in PE. 107) In PE فإنسب. 108) Lacking in B, C, and V. 109) In PE followed by لون البثر. 110) In PE ثقب. 111) In PE جاسئاً. 112) In PE لأنها رديئة جداً بل. 113) Lacking in PE.

الباب الثامن

1) Lacking in B and V. 2) In V في. 3) In V اربعين. 4) Lacking in B. 5) In V العينين. 6) In V الفكين. 7) In V المفقين. 8) In V الساعدين. 9) In V الكفين. 10) In V الاسن. 11) In V بحركة. 12) As in note eleven. 13) Lacking in C. 14) Lacking in C. 15) In C حمس. 16) In B and C اثنى. 17) Lacking in PE. 18) Lacking in PE. 19) In V الحلان. 20) In V الصدعين. 21) In PE الودجين عرقا. 22) Lacking in V. 23) In B مآبض, in C and V مابض. 24) Lacking in B and V, in PE الغرض فى علاجها مراعاة اصول ثلاثة. 25) Lacking in B and V. 26) In PE كان لمجاوره مادة. 27) In PE تعتنى. 28) In PE

.تتداركه 29) In PE فيجب ان تتداركه. 30) In PE نخبه وأساله لصدير. 31) Lacking in B and C. 32) In V فض. 33) In V الحليب. 34) In B and C شفتاها. 35) In C شقتاها. 36) Lacking in B and C. 37) Lacking in B and C. 38) In PE إلى الأدوية. 39) In PE يورم. 40) In PE يخلط. 41) In PE يجعل فيه. 42) In PE ليأمن. 43) Lacking in PE. 44) In PE يستعمل. 45) In PE شاكل. 46) Lacking in C. 47) In PE فيعالج. 48) In PE علاج. 49) In PE المقوى. 50) In B, C, and V والذي. 51) In PE followed by موضع. 52) In PE الكندر (storax). 53) In PE سوية. 54) In PE إلطخ به. 55) In PE يرى. 56) In C عرفت. 57) In PE الدواء. 58) In V كاللحمة ارخوة. 59) In PE فإسقه السمن. 60) Lacking in PE. 61) In PE إستبان. 62) In PE فإسقه السمن. 63) In PE يتعفن. 64) In V نعما. 65) This word repeated in B, C, and V. 66) In PE words reversed. 67) In PE والقريب منه الذى لم يقيح. 68) In C قاح. 69) In C سمى. 70) and 71) In PE غور كبيرا. 72) In PE على. 73) In PE the two items are reversed. 74) In PE انفجارا and different word order. 75) In PE يعترضها. 76) In PE ينفذ. 77) In PE تفتح. 78) In PE يثقا. 79) In PE فيفصل. 80) In PE من. 81) Lacking in V. 82) Lacking in C. 83) In V بالاطيل. 84) In C followed by هو يحب المرك. 85) Lacking in C. 86) In C شمعا مقصورا ابيضا, in V شمع دراهم.

الباب التاسع

1) In C الكحال. 2) In V الارباد. 3) Lacking in C. 4) In PE منه. 5) In C مفصل. 6) In PE words reversed. 7) In PE ينقطع. 8) In PE العقب. 9) In C انخفاضا وغورا, in PE غؤر and below. 10) Lacking in PE. 11) In PE ترى. 12) In PE من. 13) In PE ممكن. 14) In PE حده. 15) In C القدر. 16) In PE بما يدخل. 17) Lacking in C. 18) In PE الرفس. 19) In PE زاغ منه. 20) Lacking in PE. 21) In PE followed by فيه. 22) In PE صار. 23) In PE مما. 24) In PE عظم. 25) In PE الجس. 26) In PE بشق عظيم. 27) In PE يقعره . 28) in C صدمهما, in PE صادفها. 29) In C منهما. 30) In V سمكة. 31) In B, C, and V يصعد. 32) In PE الذي. 33) In C علك. 34) Lacking in B and V. 35) In V انما. 36) In B برا, in C ايرا, in V بروا. 37) In C ام. 38) Lacking in PE. 39) Lacking in C. 40) In PE الأعلى. 41) As in note fourteen. 42) In PE تبرز. 43) In PE لا يقال لذلك. 44) In PE محل. 45) Lacking in PE. 46) In PE حدث معه حصر. 47) In PE وتمددهما فيعرض. 48) In PE مريان. 49) Lacking in PE. 50) Lacking in PE. 51) Item two lacking in B, and items one and two are reversed in C. 52) Lacking in PE. 53) In PE المميل. 54) In PE يتفطن. 55) In PE على المجبر. 56) In PE followed by المجبر. 57) In PE يطيف. 58) In PE فما. 59) In PE تبطئ. 60) In PE followed by من الأورام. 61) In PE الربط. 62) In PE followed by من. 63) In PE النصب. 64) In PE ضابطاً. 65) In PE followed

by أغلظه. 66) In PE ان تحل الرباطات ضرورة. 67) In PE اذا. 68) In PE واذا جاوز. 69) In PE حللت. 70) In PE و. 71) In PE ولو امكنك ان تمسيك الجبائر ولا تحلها ولو الى عشرين ولم. 72) In PE منه. 73) In PE و. 74) In B and C يموت. 75) In PE دشبذ throughout. 76) In B and C من الكتاب الرابع من القانون. 77) In PE كعظام. 78) In PE فيكفى. 79) In PE يبالع. 80) In PE الإستقامة. 81) In V القرص. 82) Lacking in B and C, in V المتحد, in PE المنخذ. 83) In PE معه. 84) Lacking in B and C. 85) In PE followed by على ما قيل. 86) Lacking in PE. 87) In B, C, and V الدماغ. 88) In PE words reversed. 89) In all اللزج. 90) In PE followed by معه. 91) In PE followed by قد. 92) In V المصافات. 93) In V and PE متوسطه.

الباب العاشر

1) In V الاسفطسات. 2) In PE سبباً. 3) In V جنيته. 4) In V المنيفة. 5) In B جرم, in C جرام. 6) In V المسثويه, in PE المدرة. 7) In V الى. 8) In B, C, and V متفرقة. 9) In V متكيفه, in PE مكثفة. 10) In B تكثيفا, in V تكيفا, in PE مكثفاً ماء. 11) In PE وزن. 12) Lacking in C, in PE حر. 13) In C followed by هو. 14) In PE الهواء منه. 15) In PE وذلك لأن. 16) In V متكاتف throughout. 17) Lacking in B and C. 18) In B and C التحليل. 19) In V انعقال, in PE followed by كثير من. 20) In V اشدت. 21) In PE

البالعان. 22) In PE followed by طبيعة. 23) In PE وإذ. 24) In PE أسطقسية. 25) In PE إثنتان. 26) In PE الإثنتين. 27) In PE followed by أغلبان ولا شئ. 28) In PE خامدة. 29) In B مقله, in V منقلة. 30) In B and C متخلخلة. 31) In PE سيالة. 32 In PE مطاوعته. 33) In PE إستحفاظه. 34) Lacking in B and C. 35) Lacking in C. 36) In PE ووجودها. 37) In B and V بالحاد, in C بالحار. 38) In V بما يتكايف. 39) In PE التخليق. 40) Underlined words on margin in B. 41) In V صرفية, in PE عنصرية. 42) In V يفيدابهما. 43) In PE حاصلة. 44) In PE الكيفيات المتضادات. 45) In PE ليماس. 46) In PE عن. 47) In C تشابه. 48) In B and C الفضول. 49) Lacking in PE. 50) In C followed by الذى. 51) In C followed by التى. 52) In C and V النداء. 53) Underlined words lacking in V. 54) In V فيتعداها. 55) This and the previous word are reversed in C. 56) In V ازيد. 57) In V ملك. 58) Lacking in C. 59) Lacking in C. 60) In V بقراط throughout. 61) In V تبيل. 62) In V العظيمة. 63) In B بهاها, in C النسب, in V بهاها. 64) Lacking in B and C. 65) In C الامراض. 66) In V تررر. 67) In V فلنسم. 68) In V الجلد. 69) In C الشرايط. 70) Sic. 71) In V and C فيرحجن. 72) Number six is missing. 73) In C preceded by نحن (?)والله اعلم وما. 74) Lacking in V. 75) Lacking in V. 76) Lacking in V. 77) Lacking in B and C.